HOMEMADE SKIN CARE

20 Homemade Vegan Recipes with body butter, masks and scrubs to make the skin softer, smoother and brighter.

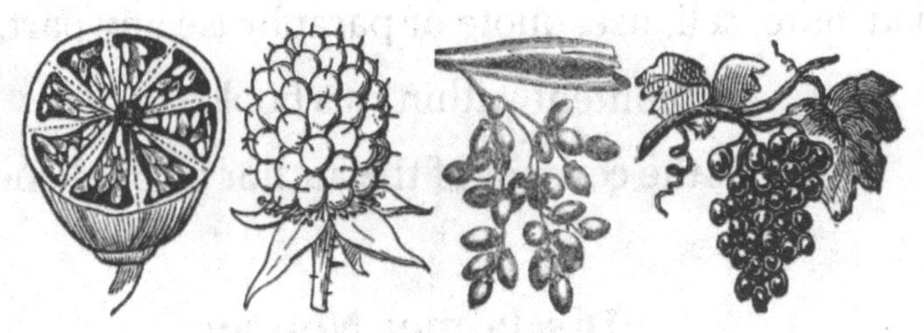

Olivia Hann

date, and reliable, complete information. No warranties of
any kind are declared or
implied. Readers acknowledge that the author is not
engaging in the rendering of legal,
financial, medical or professional advice. The content
within this book has been derived
from various sources. Please consult a licensed professional
before attempting any
techniques outlined in this book.

By reading this document, the reader agrees that under no
circumstances is the author
responsible for any losses, direct or indirect, which are
incurred as a result of the use of
information contained within this document, including, but
not limited to, — errors,
omissions, or inaccuracies.

Contents

Introductions

Everybody wants to look young with great skin and spend money on expensive beauty products that claim to have certain effects on our skin while chasing the beauty we all desire.

It's not incorrect to do so, but if there's a far better way to achieve the same or even better results on our skin just by using the right ingredients in your own kitchen, it's easy to make and cost only a few bucks, wouldn't it be great?

Popular ingredients such as an egg white, one packet of unflavored gelatin, 2 tablespoons of peppermint leaves and 1/2 passion fruit can be used to create a firming facial mask. Whip the egg white with a mixer until stiff peaks develop, then whip while sprinkling in the unflavored gelatin.

Mash the 1/2 passion fruit and add all ingredients slowly to the egg white, whipping until completely mixed. Apply 20 minutes freshly washed and rinse well with warm water.Some of you might scorn the idea of eating and putting ingredients on your face and body. But since ancient times, women knew how to use natural ingredients to beautify their skins?

One famous example is Cleopatra, renowned for her beautiful skin. She was said to use goat's milk to smooth her face.

Homemade vegan skin care recipes have many benefits. Besides being just as powerful, there's the added comfort of knowing what exactly you put on your own skin. Beauty products on the market include chemicals, additives and preservatives that can long-term adversely affect our skin.

However, you're assured of its freshness if you've prepared your own skin care recipes, as they're used right after you've made them. Your skin should benefit optimally from ingredient freshness. Use natural skin care products for your skin care scheme is also cheaper compared to shelf beauty products, so imagine how much money you can save each year.

Although there are hardly any side effects of using natural skin care ingredients, please note that sometimes you may not know which ingredient suits your skin type and may end up using one that causes you to suffer from some skin irritations if used incorrectly or you may be allergic to certain ingredients.

Another approach is to check tiny blobs inside your wrist for allergies before using it on your face or any other part of your body. You can experiment with many homemade vegan skin care recipes. If used correctly, these common ingredients from your kitchen may be your secret to safe, glowing taint.

Compared to artificially made creams and medicines, using homemade skin care products is better for the skin as they are more natural and usually healthier for delicate skin.

One of the greatest benefits you will appreciate using homemade skin care products is that you know the exact types of ingredients used when making them. You can also get all the ingredients for the drug cheaply in your local store, helping you save tons of money when you do away with pricey cream bottles or cleansers that contain artificial ingredients.

Chemicals can long-term harm your skin if harsh. Use ingredients in your kitchen, however, means that whatever you put into your skin care product is healthy and 100% natural.

This Guide discusses successful ways to take good care of your skin, along with 20 home-made vegan skin care recipes that you can start experimenting with immediately.

≪ *Thanks again for choosing this book, make sure to leave a short review on Amazon if you enjoy it, I'd be really love to hear your thoughts.* ≫

CHAPTER 1

The Business Of Skin Care

Skin is the body's largest organ. It is the primary protection against harmful microorganisms and other chemicals. Skin enables proper body temperature control. When cold, it promotes heat production. If it's dry, the skin responds by releasing heat. With these different functions, keeping skin in optimum condition is important.

This is done through a variety of skin care products on the market. There's an alternative— homemade skin care products. With a more conventional approach, certain synthetic additives cause no concerns about harmful side effects.

Here are lists of skin care recipes information that can remedy body, feet, face, and eye problems. It may help remove accumulated dead skin cells, providing a more youthful glow.

Sea Salt Body and Foot Bath

The body and foot bath offers incredible information on skin care recipes. It's one of the most affordable, easiest-to-make homemade skin scrubs.

For a soothing bath, a bowl of hot water mixes 3⁄4 cup sea salt.

Put 30-45 drops of essential oils. Use of lavender, neroli, tangerine or citrus.

Lavender is renowned for its aromatherapy.

This homemade skin care product is also a great purifier and antiseptic. Use neroli to relieve dry cracked skin. Tangerine makes the nervous system relaxing. In comparison, lemon provides a deep cleaning and revitalizing fragrance.

Once the ingredients are thoroughly mixed, the body can be easily scrubbed. Keep away from face and eyes as it is too harsh. Bathing or showering off after scrubbing. To clean the feet, just use 1⁄4 cup of sea salt and 10 to 15 drops of essential oils.

Aloe Vera Moisturizer

Aloe Vera is one of the oldest and most popular homemade skin care products. It can fight harmful microorganisms and relieve any skin irritation. This contains healing properties that can stimulate new skin cells. Problems like skin dryness or eczema will be in the past. It's definitely one of sparkling skin's homemade recipes.

This moisturizer contains fresh gel from a large Aloe Vera leaf and an extra virgin olive oil tablespoon. Mix the ingredients thoroughly. Bring on the moisturizer's light layer twice a day; once in the morning and one at night. If not used, it can be kept in the refrigerator. Preparation can last up to three days.

Potato Under Eye Treatment

Dark circles under the eye and eye puffiness were many people's problem. They desperately find ways to treat it, but some products don't deliver. This procedure contains information on skin care recipes to eliminate the problem. A potato is packed with enzymes that can help reduce dark circles.

The main ingredient needed is ¼ cup fine-grained raw potato. Add salt and a tablespoon of any dairy product. It's butter, coffee, sugar, or sour cream. Blend ingredients before making velvety creamy paste.

Chilling is an essential step ensuring maximum efficiency. Perform this method at least one hour before using. Apply over the face, particularly under the eyes. Let it live for 10-15 minutes, rinse thoroughly.

The beauty industry is a highly profitable market. Judging by the selection and price tag, consumers can become their ultimate picture of perfection. That's of course, provided they can afford it.

Saving money on skin and beauty care products isn't the only reason you should try to do - it-yourself. Mixing your own ingredients removes the guessing game of just what you put on your face. Some natural skin and hair care products often contain synthetic ingredients that your skin may not react well.

Synthetic products also incorporate scents, dyes, and other ingredients to make the product more tactile. You're covering yourself with things you don't need. And of course, you pay for the privilege of skin-up.

Creating your own beauty products is a perfect solution for people with allergies or sensitive skin because it helps the user to control exactly with what they come into contact. It's also a great way to pamper yourself and skin while saving money and looking your best.

CHAPTER 2

Skin Care For Your Everlasting Beauty

In this chapter, I'll cover all you need to know about a good skin care regimen. I will unveil the secrets of skin care that will create a healthy, beautiful face for a lifetime. It establishes, encourages and strengthens a solid basis for amazing looks and healthy skin.

I must first reassure you that understanding your skin is the first step towards a perfect, healthy skin. Without this awareness we can't pick the right skin care regimen.

There are four general skin types: dry, usually manifested by fine pores, and tends to develop early wrinkles; and is exactly the opposite, with extra shine and dilated pores, but without proper skin care routine.

It can develop acne, blackheads, and other problems; normal skin is the perfect dreamy skin with a balanced degree of hydration; sensitive skin is not that uncommon, and it can lead to serious skin problems where you least want them.

This type of skin looks reddish, it may itch, peel, and feel really tight. Eventually, blend skin that blends one or several skin types in various parts of the face on the "T" region (front, nose and shin).

Our sweat constantly expels many toxins from our bodies. Once our sweat water dries, we're left with those toxins. Such accumulate over time, weakening and drying our bodies.

To remove eye and mouth makeup, we need a makeup remover that has the same hydration as tears. Due to lack of hydration, the skin around eyes and mouth is more susceptible to wrinkles.

When making up, don't rub your eyes and ears. Just use gentle, slow movements to avoid wrinkles. Finally, use a skin-type product for the rest of your face. Apply the cleaner for a minute or so to prevent wrinkles. Several homemade face cleaners are: Milk Cleaner lemon and yogurt, Strawberry milk cleaner, etc.

Without a tonic matching your skin type, a good skin care regimen cannot be complete. The tonic extracts chemicals and debris from your skin, leaving it healthy. Tonic non-alcohol is preferred.

Alcohol-based products can cause more skin problems because they can give you a false impression of regulating your skin's oil, but actually can create even more, creating more excessive acne and oily skin. Applying the tonic over very clean skin is very important to get the full benefit. Some popular tonics are: rose water, chamomile tonic, etc.

Our skin is constantly changing, creating new and young cells everyday. These will replace the dead cells, but to enable those new cells to achieve the higher regeneration point, we must get rid of our dead ones.

Therefore, exfoliating our skin, the next step in our skin care regimen is so important. When we don't exfoliate, we have those dead cells blocking the way to the new cell, giving our skin a dark, opaque look.

Exfoliation gets rid of dead cells, leaving new ones free to rebuild the skin and maintain a youthful appearance. This rejuvenating effect is the natural result of getting rid of dead cells while stimulating young and new cell production.

Moreover, with good exfoliation, skin treatments will have better absorption and work even better at a deeper level. Many homemade exfoliators are: lime, salt, etc.

Let's think about a good skin care mask. Incorporating this into your skin care regimen will boost your skin's beauty; it will help prolong and support your skin's health and look. Using the mask continuously, the face will recover firmness and diminish wrinkles. To optimize its effectiveness, exfoliate before using masks. It makes the mask penetrate better and work at the skin's molecular level.

Warm the mask in your hand before applying it, so it will work better. Protect the eye area, there are eye-specific masks.

Through following these simple tips, you'll still experience your favorite mask's best. Many DIY masks with: clay, egg, etc.

Let's hydrate! After pampering your skin, it's essential to hydrate it. Environmental hazards and aging can change collagen production. This causes loss of hydration, giving your skin a dry, dull and unhealthy look. Luckily, finding a good moisturizer to complete your skin care regimen solves the problem.

The function of moisturizer is to keep water molecules and form a protective shield that avoids water evaporation. If we feel our skin still feels tight and dry, it means you need more water and it's time to use the replenishing serum.

These are extra skin hydration, it's more watery, and the skin should absorb it completely. Some of my preferred homemade moisturizers are: coconut, honey, etc.

CHAPTER 3

Why Choose Natural Skin Care Recipes

Let's say, the ones you can make at home are certainly a step above most of what you can buy at the store to treat your skin. The use of all natural compounds in skin care benefits tremendously because the skin comes with a host of antioxidants, essential fatty acids and a host of other vital nutrients. Without these elements, the skin can't.

The drawback with using natural ingredients that you combine in your home's comfort is you're limited to what you can use. You can take advantage of many different juices and oils, and they certainly help your skin. Though, you won't be able to get the protein complexes, waxes, and different extracts you need to complete skin healing.

The reason people turn to home-made skin care recipes is either because they are sick of the formulations that did not give them results, or they finally realized exactly what was in most of the creams and lotions sold.

The products widely used to produce such cosmetics can do little or nothing for your skin, and the truth is that a large number of substances can have a detrimental effect on your health.

There are thousands of harmful or carcinogenic chemicals used daily in cosmetic product development. As chemicals are absorbed into the skin, they gradually reach the bloodstream.

Once these harmful ingredients start traveling through your body, they reside in your organs and soft tissue. They will continue to accumulate in your tissue as long as you continue to use it.

So, you can use homemade skin care recipes much safer than the basic over the counter product, but as I noted, they'll be of limited use to you. What I'd do, instead of depending on concoctions I made at home, is simply finding one of the few companies that make 100% of all natural products. There are some fine formulas that will give you amazing results.

A line of formulations produced by a New Zealand company is becoming known as the most effective anti-aging products anywhere. Such creams contain ingredients including Manuka honey, avocado oil, and Functional Keratin protein fusion.

All of these substances are known for their ability to significantly increase skin firming tissue. Phytessence Wakame kelp extract and grape seed oil help boost skin tissue and polymer levels by preventing enzyme-degradation.

Don't mistake that. Just don't get ingredients like Phytessence Wakame and Functional Keratin for your home-made skin care recipes. Heck, even Manuka honey must first become a powder before it can be used on your skin. You should think about investing in the goods that contain these ingredients, because they can do what you can't do on your own.

Have you taken time to check your facial mask ingredients?

You could do more facial harm than good with some of the creams, moisturizers, silicone facial mask, and toners in your routine skin care regimen.

Most of us just don't give our faces a second thought, but maybe we should be more conscious. You'll see words you can't pronounce on the packets, and most of them cause allergic reactions in people.

Most will contain chemicals releasing formaldehyde and coloring related to fatigue, headaches, nausea, and asthma. All these compounds are ingested into your bloodstream as if you had consumed them. Surely there's a better way to keep our skin smooth, shiny, healthy and beautiful than by harsh chemicals.

<u>It's not the money!</u>
We used to choose personal skin care products so beautifully fragrant and packaged that we think they will have the same effect on our skin. The companies that produce these products actually pay more to sway our senses than to make our skin healthy.

Day by day, more of us see the harmful effects of some of these skin care products and make wiser decisions about our skin, our health, and the atmosphere we live in.
We give up the scent and fancy packaging for recipes, soaps, scrubs and skin care products that are completely safe for our bodies and the world around us.

You will find that commercial natural skin care products are sometimes more costly than their counterparts, but the long-term effects on your face and skin are well worth using all natural products.

The best facial masks and skin care recipes come from your kitchen. By using all natural ingredients like honey and yogurt, you get the best possible facial masks without any chemicals at a fraction of the commercial product cost.

Don't know where to start your own recipes; just search Google. You'll find enough facial mask and skin care recipes to last the rest of your life, and they'll be cheap and safe.

Recipes will be simple, using common kitchen ingredients. Recipes of fresh vegetables, oatmeal, sugar, milk, just to name a few.

Just be mindful that some women have allergies to foods like honey, milk, or eggs. When you know you can't eat some of the ingredients of a particular recipe, you shouldn't put them on your face either.

If you find one recipe that doesn't work so well for your facial recipe, just move on to the next until you find the one with the most skin benefits.

People put a lot of faith in the effectiveness of the homemade natural skin care remedies they hear about, but the question is, they are as effective as many sources claim.

Magazines and websites online always offer recipes for various mixtures they say will do wonders for your skin, and folks love the idea that their anti-aging products will cost them virtually nothing. Sometimes you get what you pay.

People turn to these formulas not only because of the money they save, but also out of disappointment with the formulas they used for counter-skin care. Cosmetic companies tend to supply us with products that don't live up to their efficacy promises, and they often contain a bevy of unsavory ingredients. Some of the ingredients in these cosmetics can actually harm you, so you must be careful what you buy.

Homemade, natural skin care anti-aging formulations are definitely safer than the counter formula norm, as they are usually packed with chemicals.

They won't offer you more benefit than the formulas purchased from the store. By using the ingredients these recipes are generally recommended to give your skin antioxidants and some essential nutrients.

Not that I'm saying that providing vitamins, minerals and essential fatty acids to the skin isn't extremely beneficial, and antioxidants are an absolute must for healthy skin.

Antioxidants can help keep you healthier by undoing the damage done by free radicals stealing electrons from the skin's chemical structures. I say, there's more to do if you want firmer, smoother skin.

You lose collagen, elastin, and hyaluronic acid at an ever-increasing rate due to enzyme activity that breaks down these substances. The development of collagen and elastin also plummet, and there's practically nothing the home-made natural skin care can do about it.

Use avocado oil to stimulate collagen growth will aid slightly, but you need more important components than this material alone.

CHAPTER 4

Benefits Of Making Your Own Organic Skin Care Products At Home

Despite the rising cost of skin care products and the high price of organic skin care products, more people are learning to make their organic lotions, creams, and soaps at home for a fraction of retail costs.

You can learn to make your own products at home with the purest ingredients available by following some simple steps, and you'll know how pure you've chosen them.

Buying Ingredients for Homemade Organic Skin Care Products First, consider the products you already use or want to use, and make a wish list of ingredients. Then go online and search for organic skin care product recipes online and choose those that appeal to you and meet your needs.

Buy the ingredients in your recipes, either at your local shopping store or online. Buy the best organic ingredients and follow the recipes closely to make sure your products are exactly what you want them to be.

Without breaking the bank, you can make use of high quality ingredients, because making skin care products at home makes them far more affordable than retail versions.

Before you start, make small batches of each product to try out which formulas, which combinations work best for you. That way you'll spend less, and if you make a mistake, it won't be a huge loss.

Start making singe batches of your base product until you add different ingredients or scents. Split the foundation into smaller batches to test each with different ingredients. Here's the best way to find the combination you prefer without wasting excess product.

Keep a notebook with the quantities and amounts of each product you use while playing with batches. You don't just want to duplicate a recipe you've already tried, you'll want to refer to your list of ingredients and measurements when one batch turns out so well, you want to replicate it down the road.

It might be difficult to prepare your own skin care products to compete with those on the shelf judging from all the hyped skin care product ads for the items we see on the shelf,.

Such ads try to make you believe they use obscure science project-based products only available to skin care firms. I'm here to tell you that making good skin care products is sometimes easier and more effective than purchasing them at your favorite drugstore.

The first thing you need to make a skin care product is a great recipe. You will find plenty of recipes online or get them from authors ' books that researched and prepared these items themselves. Many recipes are easy as mixing and mixing ingredients in a cool dry spot.

The shelf-life can be very good for natural products. This often depends on whether you use food-based or herbal ingredients. The shelf life can vary from days to months.

Having your own skin care isn't just about natural ingredients. You can also shop some of your favorite department store brand products. Such recipes are for the same operation as your favorite brands. Sure, it can make you more effective than your favorite brand.

<u>How's that, ask?</u>

Well, you can control how much active ingredient your home-made product contains. You would be surprised how many products contain just one minute of the active ingredient, yet you can see some results.

Skin care firms do this to save money by supplying their goods to the manufacturer, wholesaler, and retailer. By buying the product over 1000 tons. It leaves little room for measurable component concentrations.

If you buy this active ingredient and create your own skin care product, you track the desired results. And let me say it's amazing! You're not only getting great results, but incredible savings. Since these products are readily available from online sources, a comparable store-bought brand top product can be saved between 75-90%.

Hair abounds naturally. This even better suits natural oils and lubricants than cosmetics containing petrochemicals and artificial substances. Additionally, skin is the primary excretion organ, eradicating body waste through pores. Hair beats natural components of air, wind and rain every day. Skincare is your skincare.

Skin needs more help to stay healthy as we grow older. Natural skin care is skin care using naturally derived ingredients with natural additives, preservatives, surfactants, humectants and emulsifiers.

Natural skin care should suit your skin type. Natural skin care goes beyond including skin products. It also requires a systematic approach to treating one's body holistically. A skin care product is better absorbed into the skin than, say, mineral oil.

Those using natural skin care products are less interested in improving fake beauty, as they believe natural beauty is good beauty. Natural products made from vegetable or fruit extracts may be toxic.

Honey's antioxidant and microbial properties.

Honey's ability to maintain and conserve moisture has been recognized and used in skin care procedures as they help protect skin from breaking sun rays and rejuvenating damaged skin.

Jojoba's normal skin care.

Honey is a great skin care product to clean hair. Use a wet wash cloth to clear the pores. Once you've done that, put honey on your face like a mask. Leave it on for about 10-15 minutes and wash your face with warm water to close the pores.

Ideal for skin washing and moisturizing.

Take some pure yogurt in a tub. Then add the mixture to your face for about ten minutes to wash it off using warm water.

The skin is silky soft and smooth again. The best thing is to keep the skin looking smooth. One skin-friendly cure is not honey.

Instead of lime and cucumber.

Slice the cucumber with some squeezed lime. When assembled, add three drops of rose water. So apply the mixture and wait thirty minutes. First, wash your face with cold water and see your skin become smoother and cleaner.

Such recipes are for items that can be made in your home's convenience, where you can find all the ingredients from your local stores. Homemade products are all natural and contain no additives. Using these tips for beautiful skin, you can quickly get your perfect skin.

Jojoba's natural moisturizer.

Perhaps oil to the normal sebum. Skin soothes occasionally. Using a moisturizing cream on body skin can be helpful, especially when mature skin tends to dry. High-end beauty boutiques and e-tailers will make shea butter in many drug stores.

Shea butter is also the staple of African pharmacology due to its healing power. Also today, clinical trials indicate shea butter's ability to deliver positive medicinal results and safe, natural skin care. Oils often used in gels and soaps to nourish, stimulate and hydrate skin and hair.

Dark, leafy green vegetables are a great source of zinc and iron for healthy skin. Iron brings enough oxygen to the skin, so zinc is a perfect pimple attacker. Citrus fruits are popular components that enhance skin growth.

CHAPTER 5

Needed Tools And Ingredients For Making Homemade Skin Care Recipes

Retaining the youthful look we have always cherished since time immortal. First, it was the prerogative of kings and queens; as evidenced by the archeological excavations of ancient civilizations around the world.

Everybody today, regardless of their social level, needs a skin that is shiny, youthful and comfortable throughout their lifetime and does everything possible to achieve it.

A quest always ends with the many stores selling commercial facial products like creams, masks, and soaps. But mostly such products are so full of chemical ingredients that they harm their skin more than good.

The best way to avoid this is to go for many home-made skin care products that you can easily do with items readily available in your kitchen. Such procedures make your skin look radiant and balanced.

There are simple things to keep your home-made skin care routines. Olive oil, lemon, aloe vera gel, water, washcloth and knife.

To start facial treatments at home, wash your skin first.

Take 1 tbsp. Olive oil, usually present in every kitchen and smooth over your skin. The great thing about olive oil is that it doesn't clog the pores of the skin, but helps bring out the impurities in your skin. Such impurities trigger many breakouts and blackheads you often see in your face.

Besides the impurities, olive oil also helps make your skin smooth. Now, massage the oil on your skin for 5 minutes. Shake vigorously, but use gentle but firm motions. Use a circular motion to skin this perfect, protective oil.

Take a washcloth for your home-made skin care routine and steam it to make it hot. Make sure you're not too dry, but just comfortably hot handle. Place this washcloth over your face, massaged with olive oil, and leave until the washcloth cools down. Use this cooled washcloth to clean off your skin's excess oil.

Now take a lemon, another thing readily available, and break into two. Rub these freshly cut lemon halves over your skin.

The reason for this step of home-made skin care is to kill all the bacteria present in your skin with the lemon juice as it is a natural antiseptic. Eventually, brush around 1/2 tsp of aloe Vera gel over skin.

Aloe Vera is an outstanding natural moisturizer that helps to reduce redness often seen in most skins. To get this treatment's full benefit, make sure you do it twice a day.

Finding good-quality skin care products that don't damage your patina and keep you looking fit and healthy is often a challenging task-and definitely costly.

Cosmetics companies ensure that they keep their prices high for their goods, often a harmful and dangerous combination of chemicals that can damage the skin just as much as it tries to benefit. For skin care, homemade is definitely the best.

Every day our body sheds from its surface dry flakes, and their number increases when using artificial chemicals. By using ingredients found in nature, little of the serious harm can be caused by using synthetic chemicals products.

The average person's kitchen or medicine cabinet often holds the secret to flawless looks of great quality, with only a smattering of ingredients easily combined to yield glossy results.

The only initial outlay is optional, unlike conventional make-up products: if you can reuse your conventional health products kitchen equipment, then great.

Otherwise, you may need to buy items such as measuring spoons of different sizes to measure your ingredients; a good whisk for mixing ingredients; plus a funnel, strainer or sieve, a glass eye dropper (also called a pipette) that is used to bring in essential oils to add smells to products; a glass measuring cup that is microwave safe; a collection of small kitchen scales that can certainly be fouled.

A wide variety of items can be made from natural ingredients at home. Products like milk, olive oil, sugar and honey are often used in commercial products that you pay for in large amounts.

Face masks, spot creams, moisturizers and any number of other things several people find important to their everyday care routine can be made for a fraction of the price by following simple foolproof recipes.

Lip balms, eye shadows, and blushers can also be made from natural ingredients in any home's kitchen or bathroom. Alternatively, in nearly countless stages, there are other ways to ensure homemade skin care.

Anyone with an internet connection and an interest in moving away from the grasp of large manufacturers can also produce bath salts and crystals, as well as milk and bathing lotions. It's no longer a niche job: it's certainly mainstream.

CHAPTER 6

Homemade Skin Care Facial Masks

Making the first impression is critical. Therefore, taking good skin care is important as the face is the first body area people see when they first met you. Good facial treatment, though, is what most people fail to do. There are many (costly) product types on the market that even the most dedicated skin-care fanatic is puzzled.

It doesn't have to be boring or pricey to have good skin-care regime, like washing, toning, moisturizing and masks. Homemade facial masks are easy to make using readily available ingredients in the pantry or fridge. This makes the entire skin care process affordable and simple.

The strawberry mask refreshes and removes impurities from the skin. To make homemade strawberry mask, blend 1/2 cup ripe strawberries with 1/4 cup cornstarch. Apply to your face and leave for 30 minutes. Evite eye regions. Rinse off.

Blend one ripe peach and one white egg for homemade peach pore tightener,. Add 30 minutes to your forehead. It's a natural way to close the face's open pores.

Orange Oily-Skin Mask

Orange skin mask is highly effective in removing excess skin oil and enhancing complexion. Squeeze orange inside a bowl and add flour to make thick paste. Spread over your forehead. Then shower off for 20 minutes.

Avocado Mask

Avocado re-hydrates the skin. It's nice to apply this mask when the weather turns dry and windy. Mash a ripe avocado with olive oil. Apply to face.

The above masks are just a few of the hundreds of masks you can make at home. Some widely used mask ingredients include pineapple, cucumber (for clarifying and calming properties), natural yogurt, apple (for potassium) and oatmeal (smooth skin).

This may sound funny, but one of the advantages of using homemade facial masks in your skin care routine is — you know what you put on your face. Determining which ingredients are included in buy-over - the-counter products and the skin's response to these items is difficult. They're also high.

You should change the recipe for homemade masks if they aren't skin-fitting. But this isn't so for items' bought from shop.' If your skin reacts negatively to these products, it's a waste of money because you can't use them anymore, or you have to give them to your friends or family.

Another benefit of homemade skin care masks is its variety. Having different homemade masks is cheaper and easier than purchasing different beauty products!

Hold these skin care tips in mind. Taking care of your face needn't be expensive. It's relatively easy. Just a walk to your fridge will give you the smooth, hydrated, clear skin you like!

What ingredients will you bring in?

There are 3 factors to consider. What's your skin?

Is it dry, sticky, prone, natural or mixed?

If you're hot and humid, less oily recipes might match you. You also need to use the recipes correctly.

Once you've mastered making your own recipes for face masks, you can feel the essence of your heart. At first, however, stick to some tried and tested recipes to begin to understand the ingredients.

Using recipes with oatmeal for cooking.

Cleanse gently without drying the face. Use milk-mixed oatmeal and gently massage your face, including upward strokes. Rinse with warm water.

Banana isn't just full of antioxidants, it's a perfect gentle moisturizer. Add 1 egg yolk; 2 tsp almond oil and 1 ripe banana to make your first facial mask. Apply 15 minutes and rinse with warm water. Pat dry, clean towel.

Honey in your home masks will help retain moisture while enjoying its anti-oxidant, anti-septic and antibiotic properties. Avocado is another great moisturizer in a recipe for facial masks.

Oily Skin

Try this recipe for people with oily skin.

- **1/3 cup of cocoa;**
- **3 tbsp of heavy cream;**

- **1/3 cup of papaya, ripe;**
- **¼ cup of honey, raw and**
- **3 tsp of oatmeal powder.**
-

Directions

Blend together and apply for 15 minutes. Rinse with warm water and dry towel hold. The great recipe is 1/2 cucumber; 1 white egg; 1 tbsp lemon juice and 1 tsp basil.

Mix foods in a fridge for 10 minutes. Login and take 15 minutes. Rinse with hot water, spray with cold water.

Sensitive skin

Honey has excellent antiseptic and antibiotic properties. Mix with yoghurt for a calming mask. Try mixing 1 part organic cider vinegar with 3 parts water to make a great skin toner.

Dilute if it's too powerful.

Helps prevent acne problems. Apply aloe vera to honey for another facial mask curing recipes. Cold-pressed avocado oil is a good skin moisturizer. Clearly, if you have sensitive skin, doing a patch test first will not worsen your problems.

This is the tip of home remedies iceberg for different skin types. When you know how simple it is and how much money you can save while maintaining your skin, I think you'll be converted to try your own face mask recipes.

CHAPTER 7

Preventive Measures To Keep Your Skin Look Good

You had the skin your mother gave you before the age of 25. You've got the skin you gave yourself after age 25. Proof of the truth can be seen in the faces of people around you in this skin care mantra. Many women enjoy vivid, radiant skin until the mid-twenties. Nevertheless, as the thirties pass, the skin loses its elasticity and strength.

Luckily, you may take certain preventive measures to keep your skin look good. In addition, other items (such as the deep pore cleansing device from Clarisonic) will help to expose the most radiant skin.

Make your skin care doses below a part of your daily skin care routine to see radiant skin during the coming decades. On the other hand, you can keep your skin from looking tired and wrinkled when you grow old by avoiding such harmful skin treatments.

Wear sunscreen. Skin Care Do Wear Sunscreen. Everybody loves feeling the warmth of the sun on the skin, but note UV rays can lead to wrinkles, sunflowers and even skin cancer. Take care of your skin by sunscreening, even if only for 20 minutes, while you expect to be out in the sun.

Apply sunscreen to the face, arms, neck and hands as a minimum, as the skin on these areas is usually most UV sensitive. A

You have balanced foods to eat. In Defense of Nutrition, the book by food writer Michael Pollan urges readers to "Eat Food. Not too much. Just vegetables." The easy, nutritious philosophy of Pollan's diet is definitely good for your own skin.

Fruit and vegetables are a shock full of antioxidants, or specific chemical compounds that break up free radicals in the body that cause cancer.

Free radicals also damage the skin's cells. Including colorful vegetables and fruit with all foods for safe skins from inside, and particularly to ingest plenty of vitamin C, E, A and beta carotene.

Get plenty of water to drink. Toxins are filtered out of the water and circulation is increased. Every day, you drink 64 ounces (8 glasses) of water to keep your skin smooth and dry.

In fact, when you know that your water levels are low, it's nice to have several convenient moisturizing items in hand for that period. For instance, you might find that your cuticles dry after a night of heavy drinking and cause painful, unstinting hangnails. This is an indicator that other parts of dry skin that need a little TLC.

Instead of buying a whole shelf of individual moisturizers for such occasions, it's safer to have a couple of items that will refine your skin every time.

For instance, a drug such as Smith's original Rosebud Salve can be applied to dry lips, minor burns and rough skin patches like knees and elbows. Perhaps best of all, Rosebud Salve can be easily maintained whenever a skin care emergency occurs, since it's packed in a small round jar.

Use eye cream.

The skin around your eyes is one of the delicate and sensitive skin on your whole body. Take care of it (and stop the story crow's feet!) using the cream of your everyday skin. If you are looking

for a suggestion, please consult the Un-Wrinkle Eye by Peter Thomas Roth, which market trials in only 28 days have shown lower wrinkles up to 72 per cent.

Don't smoke

If you need to give up, just take some time to look at long-term smokers ' bodies. Yellow, papery skin with lots of wrinkles around your lips-that's what smoking gains.

Do not skimp on moisturizer.

Humidified skin is comfortable skin. In reality, you will find that your skin can spontaneously collapse just after applying a moisturizer, often enough to fill up the irritating wrinkles.

Apply a moisturizer, if your skin is still moist from shower or bath, to keep your skin healthy throughout the day. Body oil is particularly luxurious for your skin to moisturize.

Don't be erratic about your treatment for your skincare.

Cleanse and moisturize the skin regularly to compensate for ozone, and other toxins. Regardless of the skincare products you use, use them faithfully. A five-minute commitment in the morning and five minutes in the evening will make a big difference for your skin throughout your life.

CHAPTER 8

Essential Steps for Your Skin Care Routine

Face and skin are the first things people see. We want a clean, shiny, beautiful face when we leave our homes.

Unlike other skin areas on our bodies, facial skin is always atmospherically exposed and therefore easily damaged by sun exposure, chemicals, contaminants and pollutants. It is not only very important to maintain healthy facial skin, but also to prevent increased signs of aging, blemishes or acne.

While most skin care products and advertisements target women, men should have daily skin care routine. Men's facial skin is likely to get unhealthy, filthy, or infected with acne, so make sure you hydrate well and clean your facial skin. Some people used the same skin care routine as young.

They found a face wash that worked and stuck with the sink. Yet our skin shifts as we age. You may need your regular face wash to keep your skin clean, youthful.

Top skin routines require 4 steps. Great skin care routine is discipline and commitment. Most people consider their regular dirt hair washing or shaving, and grime their best efforts to keep their skin in good condition.

However, other crucial steps will keep their skin young, vibrant, healthy and firm. Although all four steps are necessary to maintain beautiful facial skin, 2 of the four steps are not needed daily.

Cleaning, toning, exfoliating and moisturizing are the four key steps to best skin care routines. Before going to bed, the face should be cleaned and moisturized. The face is healthy, clean, hydrated all day and night.

Cleansing is the first step to proper skin care. Most clean or shower at least once a day. That process is critical in removing dirt, dust, grime, grease and extra skin oil. Wet the hair, then use a clean face and neck.

Massage the face cleanser slowly upwards. Rinse your face with warm water, cool washcloth, cotton wool. A water-based cleanser is the easiest way to clean the face by eliminating chemicals that can irritate the skin.

Toning is the second step in daily skin care. Often used as toner pads or towels. Facial toners are used to erase any traces on the face of dirt, grease, or leftover cleanser.

Everyday using a toner is an option, and some people may even leave it out if they think their cleaner works well enough. A good thumb rule is to use your morning facial routine toner, but keep it out of your schedule.

Exfoliation is a key part of any skin care routine, but not daily. Exfoliation should be done at most once a week to remove dead skin cells. Although the body sloughs off dead skin cells alone, exfoliating helps speed the process.

Dead skin cells can block pores and cause acne, so prompt removal of these skin cells will reduce acne. Exfoliation, however, can damage facial skin if performed too often. Normal skin cells are replenished every 3-4 weeks, and new skin cells can destroy your skin.

Perhaps notably, moisturizing. Moisturizing the skin is so important because it avoids drying out our skin, causing wrinkles or cracks, and keeps our skin healthy and radiant. Dry skin, itchy and eye-free. Extremely dry skin can cause increased skin cell death. Using facial moisturizer.

Use the moisturizer when the skin is dry, as the pores are open. Leave some moisturizer to completely affect your skin. Hydrate whenever the skin feels dry, and rituals for skin care after morning. Make sure there are no harmful chemicals, fragrances or colors to irritate the skin.

Natural skin care products should meet all needs. Natural products survive harsh chemicals and colors, which can irritate the skin, causing breakouts. Use your skin-based products. Check your forearm, earlobe, or neck before buying. You can say if it triggers annoyance.

Recall removing all make-up before beginning your skin care routine. Don't just wash away the makeup; use proper make-up removers to absolutely clean the residual face. Remember to apply sunscreen if you're in the sun.

CHAPTER 9

Common Skin Care Mistakes

There is nobody who wants dull and dead skin, so some of us spend all kinds of money on skin care products that keep our skin soft and fresh.

Although many of these skin care products actually do what they are meant to, it is because many people unwillingly fall into many of the common misunderstandings about skin care that they get the results they get from their skin care product.

The best way to care for your skin is to realize what you do not need. Find out some of the more common misunderstandings about skin care, see if you need to change your skin care routine.

1. Too many more goods is better?

It isn't necessarily no. Too many skin products are not good for the skin. Of example, too much acne therapy may lead to more serious breakdowns, and too many eye gel can irritate and burn the eyes.

Many skin care ingredients are immediately absorbed into the skin, and spread to the affected area. The lotion of the body is a little different in that it travels over the entire body, but you don't still need much; just cover enough areas without excess of the skin.

2. The sun's harmful UV rays are the leading cause of wrinkles and sun spots and skin cancer.

Forgetting to wear a 40 or higher SPF sun screen protects you against sunburn, sun poisoning, wrinkles and other problems that the sun can cause.

Ensure to re-apply the sun block once to two hours even when it is waterproof, as soon as it reaches moisture, the SPF begins to break down and you are left unprotected. A decent sunglass is also good for a long time out in the sun to shield the delicate eyes from harsh rays.

3. One of the greatest mistakes you can make in the treatment of your skin is literally the first product to be picked up without testing the ingredients. I can't stress enough how important it is to thoroughly read the ingredients of skin care products to see if harsh substances are present.

Examples such as potassium hydroxide, SLS / SLES and parabens are known as among the most toxic and dangerous chemicals in the world of skin care. Such compounds cause skin irritation, burning, inflammation and are in some cases associated with cancer.

4. Whether you apply a wrinkle cream or hydrating every couple of days, don't expect the outcome to be blown away. To be reliable, any skin care product must be kept up to its use. If this company says "Use ALL MORNING AND NIGHT," that is exactly what it does. If you want your product results, find out how it functions in your daily routine.

A simple skin care scheme will take only about five to seven minutes. A good way to apply any skin care product is directly after a shower because the pores are open and can absorb a product more quickly, making it more powerful.

5. H2O Water is the only constant necessity other than the food that all life needs on this planet. Water is important to control our metabolism correctly, to give us energy and to flush the waste body.

Drinking plenty of water every day helps to remove toxins and contaminants from the skin and bacteria that would make the skin appear weathered and dull. Start drinking more water, and in the coming weeks, I hope you will see a marked change.

And now that you can understand and do not need some of the stuff that your skin needs properly, you should be able to effectively tweak if your skin care routine begins to look better and younger.

The best things are from nature, so try and stay with all natural skin care products and trust me to thank you for your skin. Protect yourself as well as you can from the sun and be as aligned with your scheme as possible. Finally don't forget to keep water and drink, it can't hurt you at all times.

CHAPTER 10

Home Remedies For Skin Care

Over time, home-made natural skin care products can save money. More importantly, these ingredients can be developed into countless recipes to yield wonderful results, just as a salon or spa would expect.

Nature will find answers to most man-made issues, including skin conditions. Nature has provided countless plants, botanicals and oils that can be mixed for almost any skin type. There's only room in this chapter to discover others for a few widely used ones.

<u>Raw sugar and sea salt</u>: their crystals are slightly rough and suitable for scrubs to exfoliate dead skin cells. For a soft wash, mix raw sugar or sea salt (more personal preference) with olive oil or almond oil.

Ground coffee: perfect dehydrator can be used to reduce eye puffiness or cellulite appearance.

Caffeine was known to give skin extra buzz for its antioxidant activity and incredible ability to neutralize free radicals. It also helps inhibit the acne breakout enzyme. In addition, caffeine is also an anti-inflammatory agent used to treat other skin irritations.

<u>Lemon / lime</u>: provide supple vitamin C, a strong antioxidant to regenerate collagen. Using diluted lemon or lime juice to exfoliate dead skin cells and reduce sunspots or acne scars. Be careful, undiluted or concentrated lemon / lime juice can cause skin irritation.

Apple cider vinegar (raw and unfiltered version): can be used in toner and spot treatment for acne.

<u>Yogurt</u>: makes a great facial mask, nourishing and rejuvenating skin cells. Natural acids inside yogurt help exfoliate dead skin cells, exposing the youthful look below.

<u>Pineapple</u>: exfoliates skin and promotes collagen development Honey: perfect for moisturizing dry skin and calming skin irritation.

<u>Egg white</u>: facial protein. This fits well in a mask to nourish and secure skin.

Potato juice: helps reduce puffiness under and around eyes

Oatmeal: helps relieve common skin irritations like itching due to dry skin or eczema

Jojoba oil: mildew fungicide

Almond oil: great emollient and moisturizer for skin and hair. It often relieves dry skin and common skin irritations. Massage therapists also use it as carrier oil because it is not greasy and is not absorbed too easily by skin cells.

Sweet orange oil: frequently used to reduce anxiety, digestive discomfort, and sinus congestion.

Lavender essential oil: often used to relax the body and calm the mind.

Lemongrass essential oil: used in aromatherapy to clean, refresh and rejuvenate coconut oil, suitable for moisturizing dry skin and protecting hair from protein loss. Also used in other hard soaps.

Grape seed oil: perfect for skin hydration.

Many more natural ingredients are used in home-made skin care products. Research, exploration, best performance checking.

You have either been inspired to save your body money or you want to know exactly what you are putting on your skin if you ever thought of using organic skin care products.

Regardless of why, it can be a simple and fun way to look amazing and to experience your own home-made skin care. And the best thing is that you have fresh ingredients in your house.

Facial masks

The face is normally the skin most aggressive. The facial skin needs to pick me up to help me treat my exposure to sunlight, toxic compounds by maquillage, toxins and extreme purifiers. A face mask is one of the most popular home care items to purify and calm your stressed face skin.

The use and testing of various ingredients is the best way to choose which one is best suited to the needs of your skin. The result can be obtained by combining strawberries, avocados, cucumbers, aloes, yogurt or clean clay.

Using a formula you can remove the tool or just experiment from a home-made skin treatment procedure. Mix the ingredients and spread them over your face and allow to dry for about 20 minutes. Just wash away once you get high, and you're good to go.

Skin Toners

Toners are an excellent tool for enhancing your skin and make-up, and they can save you most by doing it yourself. Toners will expand your face and skin's vitamins and antioxidants.

The best thing about home-made products such as toners is that it can only be manufactured from a few basic components such as apple cider vinegar, aspirin crushed and water. As always, finding a good recipe will get you going and you can find appropriate alternatives later if you understand the process.

Rubbing your face with a good homemade oil-based skin care product can help moisturize and calm the skin. You can make wonderful combinations of oil in some vitamin capsules like A, C and E and blend it with essential oil or cocoon oil. Brush your face with a thin layer and let your wrinkles get hydrated.

As you can see, making your own home-made skin care products is easy and you can probably make some with the ingredients you already have in your own home. You have your own line of products to use for home skin care while searching for recipes and experimenting, so you can save money and know what you put on the skin.

CHAPTER 11

Essential Components of Any Natural Skin Care Recipe

For efficacy, a natural skin care recipe should contain absorbable proteins, antioxidants and essential fatty acids. To resolve several problems that follow the aging process, it should include specific plant oils and extracts. Here you'll learn the best ingredients.

Protein

Protein is important to build new cells and fibers. The food you eat must be present in sufficient amounts. The proteins present in most skincare products are ineffective because they cannot be absorbed. Elastin and collagen exemplify non-absorbable proteins.

Protein peptides are more easily absorbed as amino acid chains are shorter. You'll see di-peptides, tetra-peptides, oligo-peptides, and others. Peptides should be derived from natural sources including tryptophan, valine, and palm oil.

Sometimes you'll see patented formulations with several peptides. HALOXYL and EYELISS, for example, are proprietary formulas found in some better anti-aging eye serums. Active to raising bags and dark circles. Each formula comprises two peptides.

According to research, one protein keratin form is absorbable. It is extracted from sheep's wool using proprietary methods to preserve its purpose. The best natural skin care recipe should include this form of "true" keratin, as it offers many benefits including increased firmness and decreased wrinkles.

Antioxidants

Most antioxidant molecules are too large to penetrate into many layers of skin. According to scientists, one of the most absorbable is coenzyme Q10 nano-emulsion.

Coenzyme Q10 naturally occurs in the skin layers, but due to sun exposure and general aging, skin content decreases. Supplementing the coenzyme Q10 content of the skin has long been a scientific aim. For this reason, researchers needed nanotechnology.

A natural skin care formula containing coenzyme Q10 nano-emulsion can minimize wrinkling and sun damage by up to 30%. It will increase collagen production in the skin, prevent free radical damage and repair damage already occurring.

Another essential antioxidant, vitamin E.

You'll find it in most skincare products, but it's not the natural form. The synthetic variety's benefits may be different. The benefits should include age reduction and a general de-aging impact.

Every good natural skin care recipe should contain plant oils like grape seed and avocado. Such oils contain vitamin E and other antioxidants, as well as essential fatty acids required to maintain the skin's moisture content. Each plant-oil benefits differently. For example, avocado oil increases collagen content in skin.

Plant extracts

Most beneficial plant extracts exist. The most useful is wakame kelp. It is the only compound believed to prevent skin hyaluronic acid breakdown, an essential compound responsible for smoothness, strength and firmness.

The typical natural skin care recipe doesn't include all the ingredients listed here. Nevertheless, the best do.

CHAPTER 12

20 Popular Homemade Skin Care Recipes You Can Enjoy

Homemade skin care can be as easy as mixing a small amount of oatmeal and milk, and making a body scrub that costs you pennies on the dollar compared to comparable grocery store products. Plus, they're fun to make, you know exactly what's going on in them, and if you have any allergic reaction, you don't have to do more than you need at a time.

Often store bought products lose their power before you can use it. You can have as little or as much as you need by making your own products. Here are some popular home-made recipes you can enjoy.

Our hands are our body's most used and seen parts. We subject them to dirt torture, harsh chemicals, and washing. We tend to forget the same care we give the rest of our body. By using a hand soak or mask, we can make our hands soft and smooth with little to no effort.

The easiest way is to soak your hands in ½ cup moist olive oil. It helps moisturize your palms, but also your hair. Another way is using a mask. Cook and mash two potatoes, add butter or olive oil and Vitamin E capsule to create the mask. Fill with the potatoes, let it dry, then rinse with warm water.

Homemade skin care products are cost-effective in this economic crisis. You can save money, but the gas it costs to go and buy new goods. And if you enjoy making these recipes, why not share them so expose your friends to the joy of home-made skin care products.

They'll thank you.

1. Exfoliating Papaya Face Mask

Fruit papaya is great for exfoliating and can help you get rid of dull-looking skin and scars with its papain enzyme.

What You Need:

- **Papaya**
- **Oatmeal**

<u>Directions</u>

1. Peel, seed, and cut into smaller pieces.

2. Place the papaya in the mixer and mix until smooth

3. Mix papaya puree in a bowl of oatmeal until you like consistency and it's easy to work with.

4. Apply the paste to your clean face, arms, or other place to exfoliate. Remove eyes and sensitive areas. Lie down and let it work 10-15 minutes before you wash it with lukewarm water.

If the face mask remains, place it in the refrigerator. Be vigilant if you have sensitive skin, and don't use it if you have a burning or inflamed skin.

2. Moisturizer, Facial Scrub, Orange Peel Mask

Moisturizing is the secret to hydrated, soft skin. You'll be surprised to know you can make your own home-made moisturizer in minutes. It definitely helps you achieve soft, smooth skin.

Ingredients:

- **Rose Water**
- **Glycerin**
- **Lemon Juice**

Directions

-Take equal parts of all ingredients and blend well.

Apply regularly before bedtime.

Keep an airtight bottle a few weeks.

3. Homemade facial Scrub

Scrubbing is another important thing that plays a vital role in a smooth, radiant face. Scrubbing and ex-foliation is very important as it extracts dead skin cells and releases new skin cells. Most natural skin care products use almond. Use almonds to make a homemade scrub.

Ingredients:

- **Almonds**
- **Fresh milk**

<u>Directions</u>

Grind almonds and blend in fresh milk to form a thick paste.

Apply uniformly and clean gently.

Clean 10 minutes later.

4. Orange Peel Mask

Oranges are a rich source of vitamin C and alpha hydroxy acid . These skin care ingredients are clinically proven to help prevent premature skin aging.

Ingredients:

- **Egg yolk**
- **Honey**
- **Orange juice**
- **Gelatin instructions**

<u>Directions</u>

Take one egg yolk and attach one tablespoon honey.

Add 1/8 cup orange juice, blend well.

Remove 1 packet of gelatin.

Mix well and add 20-30 minutes uniformly.

5. Banish Blackheads-In Style

This next blackhead mask takes a little more effort, but it's a nice treat for a herbal mask.

Ingredients:
- **oatmeal,**
- **egg white, and parsley.**

<u>Directions</u>

Boil 1/2 cup water (some water will be lost as steam).

Turn off the water at boil and add 1/3 bunch of fresh parsley or 2 Tablespoons of dried parsley for 15 minutes.

Strain the liquid to the parsley.

While the water boils, grind 2 tablespoons of oatmeal in a clean coffee grinder. If you have no coffee grinder, split the oats into pieces using fingertips.

Mix 2 tablespoons of parsley water with 2 tablespoons of ground oats for a paste.

Remove egg white, blend in a paste and run for 10 minutes.

Add a few drops of your favorite essential oil to supplement care.

We don't suggest e.g. peppermint! Lavender or other essences will fit well.

6. Almond Scrub

Ingredients:

- **1 cup of raw almond pulp**
- **Half cup cold pressed sweet almond oil**
- **3-4 drops of essential oil (using lavender in this case)**

<u>Directions</u>

- Remove pulp and almond oil until well mixed.
- Apply the required essential oil. Mix well.
- Place in cold fridge jar (place a few days).

9. Honey Wash Moisturizing

Ingredients:

- **1 tablespoon oat or rice bran**
- **1 tablespoon honey**
- **1 teaspoon cream**

<u>Directions</u>

Heat gently in a microwave or stove, stir ingredients until well mixed.

7. Homemade Face Mask Recipe For Sun Damage

Ingredients:

- **Start with a fatty acid-rich base oil, like avocado oil, which also has regenerative qualities.**

- **Other oils, such as carrot seed, rose hip and walnut oils, have anti-aging and firming properties and are perfect for skin damage or maturity.**

<u>Directions</u>

Mix such oils in a base of: 2 tablespoons of either calophyllum oil (tamanu) coconut oil, or rose hip oil (use a combination of all three and in equal parts).

Apply 10 drops of carrot oil and/or sea buckthorn oil and 5 drops of avocado oil. These are both rich in antioxidants (vitamins C, A and E) with potent repair benefits

Blend these ingredients together well and apply twice daily to affected areas.

This blend can soak in quickly and help protect skin from further damage while repairing what's already done.

Do this, and within a week you'll see an increase, and a dramatic improvement over several months.

8. Firming Egg White Homemade Mask Recipe

This is a very good skin tightening and firming mask. Prepare for best results the day before.

Ingredients:

- **One whipped egg white**
- **1 tablespoon red wine**
- **3 drops of yarrow oil or bergamot oil or a teaspoon of mashed banana**

<u>Directions</u>

MIx and leave 2 hours or overnight sitting in the refrigerator if you have time.

Apply to skin in a thin layer and leave for half an hour to forty minutes. Wash warm water and add your favorite moisturizer.

10. Hydrating Cream And Avocado Moisture Mask

This is a very rich mask you can make, depending on your personal preference, oilier or drier.

Ingredients:

- **1 tablespoon of almond, olive, coconut or 1 teaspoon of avocado oil**
- **1 tablespoon of honey**
- **1 teaspoon of milk,**
- **mayonnaise or plain yogurt or one egg yolk**
- **1/2 mashed avocado**

<u>Directions</u>

Mix well, add to skin and leave for 10 minutes to half an hour. Wash your favorite moisturizer with warm water.

11. Sparkling Skin Exfoliating Scrub To Lighten Scars

This remedy removes or lightens scars and brightens the skin exposing sparkling fresh soft skin cells.

Ingredients:

- **1 tablespoon of honey**
- **1 tablespoon of brown sugar**
- **1/4 teaspoon of salt or baking soda 1 teaspoon of molasses (optional)**
- **1 teaspoon of almond meal or oatmeal finely ground (optional)**
- **1 tablespoon of almond oil with a few drops of avocado oil (optional)**

<u>Directions</u>

If you have oily to normal skin, you may attach a squeeze of lemon, lime or grapefruit juice. Then wash off for 5 minutes.

12. Homemade Skin Natural Peel Exfoliant

This remedy helps remove discoloration, smooth raw skin, and take old flaky skin off. It promotes new cell development, is rich in antioxidants that hold protective and vitamin-repairing skin. Use it weekly and you'll see smoother, radiant skin emerging.

Ingredients:
- **1 tablespoon of fresh pineapple**
- **1 tablespoon of papaya,**
- **cantaloupe or pawpaw fruit**
- **A few crushed berries (any berries are fine)**
- **1 tablespoon of crushed kiwifruit**
- **1 teaspoon of honey**
- **1 teaspoon of molasses (optional) or yogurt.**

<u>Directions</u>

Keep on for no more than 10 minutes as this is a very solid mask with active enzymes and fruit acids acting as a chemical peel. It's very strong and skin-stimulating. Use twice a week for gentle, smooth teint.

13. *Bleaching Mask for Dry Skin*

Ingredients:

- **A cup of chopped strawberries**
- **A cup of sliced cucumber**
- **And a cup of chopped apricots**

Directions

Take a cup of chopped strawberries and blend with a cup of sliced cucumber and a cup of chopped apricots. Mix in a blender to form a nice stiff paste, which you can then apply in the evenings after having your bath or shower.

Rinse with warm water for at least 30 minutes. For those with dry or sensitive skin, this is a particularly good bleaching mask, and if done regularly, it can help reduce fine lines. Freshly prepared paste can be kept in the refrigerator, so if you wish, you can prepare larger quantities.

14. Lemon Juice Bleaching Mask

Ingredients:

- **Two heaped table spoons of sour**
- **One lemon juice spoon**
- **Two olive oil spoons**

<u>Directions</u>

Combine two heaped table spoons of sour cream or unflavored natural yogurt with one lemon juice spoon and two olive oil spoons. Lemon juice is a powerful bleaching agent, so this recipe may not be appropriate in some rare cases, particularly if one has extremely dry skin.

That said, it's a great recipe because sour cream (or yogurt) and olive oil will leave your skin moist, soft, and beautifully fed.

15. Skin Exfoliating Bleaching Mask

Ingredients:

- **For this skin bleaching mask you need two heaped spoons of sour cream or plain yogurt, two spoons of good quality oatmeal, and one or two red win spoons.**

Directions

Mix the ingredients to create a good paste and apply liberally. Ideally, the mask should be used daily, at least once a week. The nice thing about this mask is it serves a dual purpose, not only bleaching the face, but also exfoliating the skin.

16. *Ultra-Dry Skin Cleanser And Moisturizer*

Ingredients:

- **½ Teaspoon grapefruit extract**
- **1 Glycerin teaspoon**
- **1 Jojoba teaspoon, Word or vegetable oil**
- **2 Once aloe vera gel**
- **4 Rosemary essential oil**
- **8 drops Sandalwood essential oil**

<u>Directions</u>

Mix all ingredients carefully before adding, and make sure the mixture is placed in a jar that you can quickly shake before use.

17 . Moisturizer

Ingredients:

- **3/4 Ounce beeswax**
- **1 Cup diluted**
- **1 Vegetable oil cup**
- **24 Lower eye lower geranium essential oil**
- **800 IU liquid vitamin E**
- **Much more complicated to make.**

<u>Directions</u>

You'll need to heat the oil and beeswax until the wax slightly melts, but it's not so hot you can't touch it.

Then you'll use a blender with the removed lid center to combine the water with the high setting oil and wax mixture until it solidifies into cream.

18. Cleanser for Oily Complexion Cleanser

Ingredients:

- **½ Teaspoon grapefruit extract**
- **1 Glycerin teaspoon**
- **1 Teaspoon vinegar**
- **2 Ounces hazel**
- **2 Cypress essential oil fall**

<u>Directions</u>

Combine all the ingredients together and apply to the face, then rinse off. Also, be sure to store the mixture carefully before each use.

19. Toner

Ingredients:

- **1 Tablespoon aloe gel**
- **1 Fall essential oil ylang-ylang**
- **3 Drops essential lemon oil**
- **Cedar wood essential oil 5 drops.**
- **2 ounces witch hazel**

<u>Directions</u>

Mix both ingredients with finger or cotton ball / swab.
Make sure the container you store your toner can shake safely
before using the drug.

20. Baking Soda

Baking soda-controls oily skin, gently extracts dead skin cells and balances the pH level of the skin

Ingredients:

- **Gel-anti-inflammatory or Aloe Vera Juice ,**
- **skin hydrator**
- **Tea Tree Oil- anti-fungal, anti-bacterial, anti-irritant preparation:**

<u>Directions</u>

Step 1-Pour around 4 oz. (1/2 cup) baking soda in a clean, small bottle of convenience.

Step 2— Add the aloe vera juice to the baking soda, stirring several drops at a time, until creamy, liquid-like paste is created. If the mixture is too watery, simply add more baking soda.

If the mixture gets too thick, simply add more aloe vera juice. Don't make the mixture too watery or too thick, enough smooth and liquid-like enough to pour into a container.

Step 3—Add about 20-30 drops of tea tree oil to the paste. Mix well then. If using a container, blend well.

Functions:

Removes pore-clogging dead skin cells Kills acne-causing bacteria Calms inflammation associated with acne instructions for use:

Simply wet face, then rub in circular motions throughout the skin (concentrating on problem areas) **for 30-60 seconds**. Rinse for elimination. Pat dry. Using 2-3 times weekly. Use on non-sensitive skin once a day if necessary.

While homemade skin care recipes are great fun, you'll want to make sure they have a little more science behind them when it comes to skin care products you use everyday.

This way you can get far more benefits, like deep moisturizing, glowing skin, and ageing signs prevention.

« Are you enjoying this book! If so, I'd be really happy if you could leave a short review on Amazon, it means a lot to me! Thank you. »

CHAPTER 13

Skin Care Recipes: Using Natural Ingredients

Our skin can handle its own bacteria environments that cannot be removed by cleaning. These bacteria keep the skin in check and have an essential part in "balanced skin."

When the balance is disrupted, an overgrowing infection can occur, eliminating beneficial bacteria, leading to yeast build-up that can cause problems like acne production. Therefore, proper care is essential to prevent such skin problems.

Many people are now confused by all these treatments that promise to make their skin look better. But cosmetics should be used carefully on the skin because it may not suit your skin type, it may just cause some trouble. Luckily, natural skin care procedures have proved to be more successful on the skin, not that difficult.

Treating your skin naturally is better than chemical cosmetics, as they may be too harsh for sensitive skin. We need to understand that skin sensitivity is important in our treatment. You can keep healthy, glowing skin, and there's no need to use makeup and waste too much of your money. Just give your skin the right natural care recipe.

Until beginning your skin care recipe, first analyze your skin type. Here are some examples of different skin types:

Normal Sensitive Oily Type

Here are simple skin care tips for different skin types:
What you need:

- **1 Apple**
- **2 Tablespoons Honey**

Direction:
Chop the apple and use a blender until you get a fluffy, smooth texture.
Add honey and combine well ingredients.
Refrigerate for ten minutes.
Apply mixture evenly on a clean face.
Leave on the face for 20-30 minutes and rinse thoroughly.

Normal Sensitive Oily Type

What you need:

- 1 mashed banana
- 1/2 cup oatmeal, cooked with milk
- 2 egg
- 1 tablespoon honey

<u>Direction:</u>

Combine ingredients together in large bowl. Apply the mixture to the face; massage it slowly and then leave for 15 to 20 minutes. Rinse warm water.

For Normal Skin Type Apple Honey Mask

What you need:

- **2 carrots (cooked and mashed)**
- **4 honey spoons**

<u>Directions:</u>
Blend the mashed carrots with honey.
Refrigerate for ten minutes.

Apply gently to the skin and leave it on the face for 10 to 15 minutes. Rinse with cool water.

For Dry Skin Type Honey and Egg Mask

What you need:

- **2 tablespoons of honey**
- **2 egg yolk**
- **1 tablespoon of almond oil**
- **1 tablespoon of yogurt**

Directions:

Mix all ingredients together in a large bowl and stir well until thick.

Apply the mask to your face for 5-10 minutes, and wash your face thoroughly with warm water and mild soap.

Some of the best DIY face masks ever produced are simple, cheap and home-made.

You will be tempted to taste the nutritious and delicious recipes designed to treat your face.

There are a few simple recipes for home-crafted face masks based on your unique skin regardless of whether you have oily, dry, allergic or mixed skin.

1. Oily Skin Face Mask

Try yogurt or a plum mask if your skin is somewhat oily or brown.

Plain or organic yogurt is a hydrate agent that allows your skin to efficiently shed dead skin cells and restore new skin cell growth, filled with lactic acid.

Plums have antioxidant vitamins A and C that protect your skin from free radicals and enhance your skin's resilience and softness. Such two different vitamins are commonly used in oil control and anti-acne skin care products.

Recipe: Poach the four mixed plums thoroughly and let them cool. Mash together a few tablespoons of plain or organic yogurt, a spoonful small of sweet amonds oil, and add only sufficient cornflour to make your face workable

Caution: This is a very sticky and messy recipe!

2. Dry skin face mask

Avocados are one of our planet's healthiest foods. This makes sense because they contain omega-6 and omega-9, the two fundamental fatty acids (which contribute to the suppleness of the skin and the regeneration of the tissue), vitamin E moisturizing characteristics and chlorophyll (the essential substance in plant life which helps our cells to regenerate). Avocados are good for dry skin as they easily absorb into the skin.

Recipe: Crush a prime advocate full. Add a small spoonful of super-hydrated liquid sweet mixture and mix them before adding.

3. Sensitive Skin Face

Butter is an excellent vitamin A source. As vitamin A helps restore skin texture to collagen fibers deep within the skin and accelerates the blood flow, it's essential to remove wrinkles and fine lines.

Recipe: Peel off a tablespoon and let it acclimatize to normal room temperature. When the butter is warm, add a little porridge oats and a sprinkle of creamy plain yogurt. Blend well the ingredients until they are smooth enough to apply easily to your face. The blend has a cool and calming effect.

4. Skin Face Mask

Bananas are a good source of nutrients that make the skin become smooth and incredibly soft when used topically. At the same time, they are perfect for mixed skin types because they are not dry.

CHAPTER 14

Homemade Skin Bleach – Easiest And Most Effective Homemade Skin Whitening Recipes

Medium, radiant, healthy skin, every woman's fantasy. To realize this vision, ladies are ready to do whatever it takes to achieve this perfect, bright complexion.

Harsh and harmful creams are often used, regardless of their long-term impact on women's health. Homemade skin bleach is sometimes ignored as the most powerful, healthy, natural way to brighten one's teint.

Unfortunately, hundreds of toxic factors threaten your skin causing a wide range of skin imperfections: air pollutants, stressful lifestyle, unhealthy dietary habits, sun damage, long-term use of dubious quality skin care products, etc. This list could go on and on.

Homemade skin bleach can be one of the best solutions to many issues, such as skin discoloration, dark circles, freckles, melasma, sun damage, birthmarks, age spots, acne scars, etc. This approach has numerous advantages.

The best part is-you decide what ingredients the skin whitening product contains. You should remove those you know are allergic to and add ingredients that will nourish, moisturize your skin, produce a gentle peeling effect to effectively double the procedure's efficacy.

Homemade Skin Bleach:

Ingredients:

- **2 table spoons of red wine,**
- **2 table spoons of light sour cream (or plain yogurt).**

Directions

Mix all the ingredients.

Shake softly and quit for 15 minutes.

Rinse with warm water.

Oatmeal acts as a gentle wash, removing the top layer of dead cells, exposing rejuvenated younger skin. Sour cream has a blanching effect. Such a routine treatment will make your teint look younger, smoother, and make small wrinkles disappear.

2. Olive oil table spoons, 2 sour cream table spoons, 1 lemon juice tea spoon.

Lemon juice has the best bleaching strength, sour scream rejuvenates the skin, and olive oil makes it fluffy, smooth and vitamin-fed.

3. Mix a few fresh strawberries, apricots and cucumbers (in equal proportions) into a thick paste and spread for about 10-15 minutes once or twice a day. This mask is perfect for dry, sensitive skin.

All skin whitening masks should be gently placed on your face along so-called "color lines": from your chin to your ears from bottom to top.

CHAPTER 15

Natural Skin Care Recipes Made With Honey

Did you know it's been around for a long time using honey as a basis for homemade beauty products? Honey, and its antimicrobial properties, is the perfect moisturizer for your skin. Honey has healing properties.

The best honey to use on your skin is raw, unfiltered, organic honey.

Here are some natural skin care recipes made with honey that will make your skin feel beautiful just in time for the holidays.

1. **Next, rinse face with warm** water and add a thin portion of organic honey.

Leave the honey mask on your face for up to 30 minutes, rinse with warm water. Final water rinse will close the pores. Use this mask weekly.

2. **Fill your tub with warm water**, then add 1/3 cup of honey and 1 cup of whole milk or cream. Soak in the tub for a relaxing honey-milk bath.

3. **For the most beautiful facial scrub** / exfoliate you've ever experienced, add 1 cup of honey, 1 cup of coarse sea salt or kosher salt and 1/24 cup of olive oil. Apply this mixture circularly to your skin, then rinse thoroughly.

4. **For a perfect after-shampoo soothing rinse**, add 1 teaspoon honey to 4 cups of warm water. Shake the mixture well, then rinse your hair. Don't clean this mixture. Dry hair as usual.

5. **If you have really dry hair**, you're going to love this. Honey's a great hair conditioner. Just blend 1⁄4 cup of honey with 2 olive oil spoons and 2 aloe vera gel spoons.

Make sure the aloe vera is pure, not aloe vera gel-containing. If you have an aloe plant, use your plant's aloe. After adding everything, work the mixture through your hair and leave for about 30 minutes. Rinse with warm water.

6. Honey-Cucumber Facial Mask

This is also a nice homemade mask. Puree a sliced cucumber with honey in a blender. Place the mixture on your face for 30 minutes, then rinse. Your skin will rejuvenate.

7. Make your own lip balm.

Honey can make your own lip balm. Only mix a teaspoon of honey with 1/4 teaspoon of coconut oil, add before going to bed. This is a great recipe for winter's cracked and sore lips.

Only pick up a jar of fresh, unfiltered, raw honey and make natural skin care recipes that your body will love.

CHAPTER 16

Natural Ingredients For Beautiful Skin

Looking beyond your own kitchen or local grocery store, you don't need to find good, healthy skin care solutions. Bananas, almond, papaya, and olive oil, oats, honey— all play a part.

These foods are packed with minerals, enzymes, and natural vitamins to make your skin look clean, clean and soft yet. No longer need to pay experts as you learn to make your own skin care treatments at home.

5 Home Remedies for Common Skin Care Problems

Below are 5 great recipes you can make at home to remedy our most common skin problems.

Prepare to easily use fruits, vegetables and natural ingredients in your local grocery store for the following procedures.

Use this simple exfoliating blend of pineapple and olive oil to dissolve the old dead cell.

Pineapple enzymes gently remove the top layer of old skin and olive oil provides well-known vitamin E skin supplement to restore smooth, supple surface.

Add 4 pineapple pieces and 3 tablespoons Extra Virgin olive oil to make a smooth paste.

Leave for 15 minutes, then wash with water.

Banish Blackheads— Blackheads certainly don't look good quickly and easily, and since we know they're the product of blocked pores, we will clean them up. Two classic cleaners to keep your blackhead-prone areas dry.

The first is a basic, two-ingredient quick-routine cleaning solution.

Combine soda with water to make a paste.

Apply 10 minutes to your nose, or at least blackhead problem areas, and let this absorbent mask wick the follicle-covering oil and debris.

Make Your Own Homemade Moisturizer

Sun dry out our skin in the summer and wind in the winter, robbing us of the youthful look. Restore natural humidity with this simple, two-ingredient recipes!

You may need to pick up some almond oil if you usually don't use it and get a good, smooth, ready-to-use avocado in store.

Use 1/2 to 1/3 of avocado to make this simple moisturizing skin mask, blend it with four drops of almond oil and leave for 30 minutes

CHAPTER 17

What Are The Most Commonly Used Homemade Face Mask Recipes?

If your skin has recently misbehaved, it is time to take a break and treat your face; what better way to spoil your skin than using facial masks. But do not yet go out to buy a facial mask, try one of these homemade facial mask recipes.

When you have acne-prone and oily skin, a home-made banana mask can be used. The banana mask consists of one mashed banana, 1 teaspoon of sweet wine and a couple of drops of lemon juice.

You should substitute orange juice for lemon juice if you have sensitive skin. Apply the mask on your face and take care of the oily regions. Keep the face mask on and then clean with water for at least 15 minutes.

Bananas are one of the fruits with the highest nutrients. It is good for the skin as it contains high amounts of potassium, magnesium, iron, iodine, zinc, vitamin A, B-complex, E, and F.

Honey helps to clear up acne because it has antibacterial and curative properties. However, it moisturizes without a greasy sensation. Citric acid is found in lemons and oranges. Citric acid is used to dry up acne and helps to lighten defects.

The green mask is another recipe for a diy facial mask. The mask consists of 1 tablespoon of green tea, 4 tablespoons of aloe vera gel and a drop of the essential sweet orange oil.

Combine the ingredients and raise the aloe vera gel if the mix is too smooth. Apply the mask to the area of your face and neck and quit for about 10-15 minutes. Wash the mask with warm water afterwards.

The green mask is one of the best recetes for face masks and can be effective for acne and other skin conditions. Green tea makes your skin wonderful. It is not only rich in vitamins C and E, but also high in antioxidants.

Green tea helps to combat free radicals ' harm. On the other hand, Aloe Vera is a great rejuvenator of skin. It also has anti-aging, antibacterial and soothing properties, apart from moisturizing. Meanwhile, the essential oil of sweet orange refills dry and damaged skin. It also helps to relieve skin irritations including eczema.

One of the recipes for facial masks, particularly for dry skin, is the mask for olive oil and avocado. The mask is made of half an avocado's flesh and is mixed with a tablespoon of olive oil. Apply the mask to your face and leave it for 20 minutes to get its full benefit. Then thoroughly rinse the mixture with warm water.

Avocado is perfect for dry skin because it contains essential nutrients such as vitamin A and vitamin B. Avocado oil is also very similar to face oil, so it hydrates the skin without a hard, gray brush. Meanwhile, olive oil is known to encourage smooth, glowing skin.

It is also a fantastic hydrator, leaving the skin dry and smooth. You should use a home recipes for facial masks using cat litter if you want a facial mask for deep cleansing. Mix four tablespoons of non-scented cat litter with warm water to make your mask. Apply the mask uniformly, leave on for 15 minutes, then rinse with warm water.

The 100% pure and unscented litter is made of bentonite clay. It is said to be the same ingredient in the facial masks made by high end beauty spas. You can now make the same masks with one of the facial mask recipes in the comfort of your home.

The same (sometimes even better) as their commercially made counterparts work homemade facial masks less the synthetic ingredients. Many of the products can be found easily in your kitchen or in a nearby store.

Another good thing about homemade facial mask recettes is that you can choose the ingredients that are perfect for your skin. However, these home-made facial mask recipes are very easy to make and much cheaper.

There are many products you can use to make face masks. In reality, if you want to make a homemade face mask, you would not normally have to buy anything. Many homemade facial mask recipes will require ingredients in your fridge or kitchen desks.

There are many recipes available for home-made facial mask recipes. What you need to find is the right recipe for your skin. While commercial and homemade facial masks are primarily used for cleaning, some are also used to treat skin conditions. Below are natural facial mask recipes for various skin types and skin problems.

Oily skin

Many people have a big problem with an oily skin. Some people may find it irritating to have a shiny face due to excess oils. If the oils have remained on your face for a long time, they can become blocked and pimples.

Home-made mask recipes are usually made with white egg, sweetheart, limon juice and yeast powder. Such products remove oils effectively. Indeed, the lemon juice alone can solve the acidity of the oil.

Dry skin

A lot of people are affected by dry skin. Apart from a hydrating agent, a home-made mask can help treat dry skin. The following ingredients are used in most homemade facial mask recipes for dry skin: honey, butter, egg yolk, and milk.

These ingredients are known to be good hydrating agents. If mixed together, a paste that can be used as facial mask can be formed. You can simultaneously clean and moisturize your skin. Cocoa or chocolate is said to be helpful in the treatment of dry skin in some recipes.

Pimple, Zit, Acne

Pimples are another big problem in the nose. Dermatologists suggest some pimples are caused by stress, while others are caused by dust and oils obstructed by pores. Home-made facial mask recipes include sweetheart, muscat, cinnamon and lemon juice.

A honey, nutmeg and cinnamon combination can take all the dirt and oils from your face and leave it pimple. Lemon juice is useful, on the other hand, since excess oils will dry on your skin. It helps to prevent further oil and dirt contamination producing pickles.

Another option is to produce a soda bakery-mix soda bakery with water. It is very straightforward, yet the solution is an effective face mask to treat and prevent zit. Ultimately, egg yolk is also the main ingredient in home-made mask recipes for acne. Egg yolk is abundant in acne treatment by vitamin A.

Big pores

Although not a serious problem, many people want pores on their faces to be tightened. Homemade face mask recetes contain milk and oatmeal for enlarged pores. Some of them also combine with lemon juice. The oatmeal tightens the pores while the milk increases the elasticity of the skin.

It is crucial that you choose the right homemade mask recipes based on the needs of your skin. It will help to manage the skin problem faster and more efficiently.

CHAPTER 18

The Best Natural Ingredients for Homemade Facial Masks Recipes

If you can make one recipe, you will be well prepared to produce your own personal product line at home. Your skin will feel healthier and look better, and your loved ones will comment on the new one.

The most important thing about making natural masks at home is to make fresh, organic skin ingredients. Furthermore, the products in your local supermarket are really easy to find.

How do you get these recipes started?

You must use fresh ingredients to make the most of it. Since most home-made remedies contain herbs, you'll want to stock your closet with fresh herbs. You may have already grown in your greenhouse.

Don't worry about buying any item you need immediately for recipes. Take an inventory of the items you already have and store them slowly in the future.

I've included a list of the most used products in cosmetics, but for your new blends, toner and facial malts, you'll also need kitchen items like a funnel, a little cockerel or strainer, as well as containers of little kind, small bottles and spray bottles.

- **Citrus fruit**
- **Dairy products**
- **Eggs**
- **Oatmeal**
- **Wheat**
- **Honey**
- **Olive oil**
- **Vinegars**
- **Tea bags**

Benefits of using natural ingredients such as above do more than mitigate the impact of the commercially made synthetic ingredients. Some common items used for home-made cosmetic include: They offer skin the minerals and vitamins necessary for radiant beauty.

Eggs

The egg is an extraordinary skin care product, from ancient Chinese civilization to modern-day celebrities. Eggs function as an emollient natural skin that acts to relax the skin. Many people who create home-made face masks have found that it works fantastically to reduce acne, redness and inflammation, making it a perfect addition to natural face dishes.

Honey

Is it true that your skin has a natural sweetness? Totally! Absolutely! Honey helps to preserve the natural skin acid. It also provides the essential enzymes for balanced vitamins and minerals in addition to natural sugar. The rich amino acids enhance the skin's appearance over time. It also serves as a good cleanser.

You can make your own home-made face masks recipes now that you know more about the benefits of natural ingredients. Find out more about combining ingredients that help your skin type and avoid allergic ingredients. Such ingredients are easy to find and will greatly benefit your skin's appearance.

CHAPTER 19

The Magic of Oils For Skin Care

If you have odious skin nothing is more important than good natural skin care. While dry skin needs extreme humidity, those with oily skin suffer from excessive moisture like oil and the problems involved. The good news is that normal, oily skin care will solve these problems.

The lack of signs of aging as well as dry skin is one of the commonly overlooked benefits of fatty skin. This is because the oil drums have extra moisture. Treatment for fat skin combines the anti-aging benefits of fatty skin with the removal of excess moisture. Fat skin treatment will also make your skin beautiful.

Oily skin patients also need washing of their faces and are typically prone to acne. Overactive oil glands can lead to acne if proper care for the oily skin is not taken. Grime and debris collect quickly on oily skin and block pores, which promote bacterial growth and acne development.

Through washing your skin oily you can help prevent acne through removing excess oil. Cleanse the skin of carbon and warm water ingredients for the best results. A natural cleanser removes dirt and grime and performs miracles on oily skin.

Upon washing, clean your face with warm water and then apply a toner or an astringent made from a natural ingredient recipe. Excess oil can be absorbed by natural toner without changing the pH of your skin or losing your essential moisture face.

Natural oily skin care with natural ingredients is much safer than using tough, skin irritating substances. Chemical products for skin care can often lead to a severe oily skin condition called Seborrhea.

For lack of skin moisture, seborrhea produces oil under the skin surface through the use of artificial skin care products that are dry. The top layer shrivels due to the oxidation of the chemical skin care product.

This prevents oil from flowing from oil glands, blocking pores and causing acne. Natural oily treatment of skin made from natural ingredients is good for oily skin and helps prevent Seborrhea infection.

To people with oily skin who are also scaly, an oily skin scrub made from natural ingredients should be used. A natural scrub exfoliates your skin by removing essential moisture.

Another great option for oily skin care is a natural facial mask. Excess oil is covered gently with natural clay masks. Apply a natural mask with the natural ingredients of a recipe, and rinse with warm water. A moisturizer is then applied with natural oily skin treatment.

Experiment with natural skin care by making your own oily skin care products home with recipes and natural ingredients. Through playing with various recipes, you can find the natural ingredients that work best for your fat skin. The more ingredients and recipes you are using, the better the natural oily skin treatment.

One of the main differences among classical skin care and natural or organic skin care is that they are not "solid" ingredients, such as green tea or vitamin c, that account for up to 5% of products, but the fundamental ingredients.

For natural skin care, the essential ingredients are often a mixture of vegetable oil with butter or wax, rather than traditional skin care synthetic ingredients. The use of essential oils greatly helps the skin.

Fundamental oils contain nutrients including vitamins, minerals and essential fats, which help and cultivate the skin rather than be an inert synthetic carrier for the active ingredients. I would go to mention essential oils as active ingredients in skin care.

Furthermore, up to 95% of all natural ingredients have a protective "aging" effect on the skin. In comparison, the synthetic basic ingredients in modern skin care have no major therapeutic benefit.

Many factors affect the absorption of topical ingredients into the skin and, in addition, many topical creams only lie on the surface of the skin, effectively plumping skin cells into their surface.

The skin is highly absorbent and relatively permeable to fats soluble and water-soluble. Fat soluble ingredients like oils are absorbed more quickly to feed the skin and have better effect on the cell membrane and the skin matrices.

Instead of having a' top' effect, oil can also hold essential oils, phytonutrients, vitamins and minerals in the skin as carriers. Oils also help to avoid skin dehydration by providing an effective barrier to water loss, leading to more hydrated plumber.

That carrier oil is absorbed by viscosity or thickness with thicker oils which tend to penetrate the skin slowly. Fine light oils can be used on the face in general as they absorb quickly and easily penetrate the skin without feeling grateful. Heavier oils are ideal for dry skin, skin on the body, like bath oils and massage oils.

The degree of unsaturation also influences oil absorption. The polyunsaturated fat the higher the absorption the oil produces. The Rose hip oil is high in polyunsaturates and has a fairly low viscosity, suitable for use in the face serum or cream, because it absorbs easily into the skin.

Cold-pressed oils are more unsaturated than heat-extracted oils and are therefore preferable. Cold-pressing involves putting the noodle or seed into an "expeller" that dries out the oil.

Any heat generated by friction does not harm the oil or its components. Heat extraction requires up to 200 ° C temperatures, which dramatically increases oil yield, which makes it much more profitable but also destroys oil nutrients.

High temperatures destroy unsaturated fatty acids easily and therefore heat extracted oil levels are significantly lower. While these oils are widely used in cooking oils, the medicinal effects of the cold-pressed variety should be avoided for use in the skin and aromatherapy.

A common misconception is that adding oils on the skin only worsens oily skin and creates more congestion. Heavier oils may be placed on the skin surface longer before absorption, which is not suitable for oily skin. Nevertheless, the smaller, less viscous oils are consumed very easily and often do not contribute to the balance oils for the skin.

Instead of being on the surface layer, the oils are easily absorbed into the skin and are unlikely to cause or exacerbate irritation. However, waxes and butter are the basis of many natural skin care products.

Although they are extremely beneficial to the skin, they are more likely to be on the surface and are therefore more likely to contribute if there is already a problem of pollution. These are unlikely to cause irritation that has not existed in the past and the skin response depends on the type of skin.

The ratio of waxes to butter to oils in different skin types varies. If you are unsure of which substance to use for your skin type, the manufacturer or supplier will be most suitable for your skin type.

There are great deals of healthy carrier oils used both in skin moisturizers and serums and the variety of natural products available which are that with nutritious base oils. Various oils are appropriate for various types of skin, so knowing some basic facts about base oils allows you to find the best drug for your skin.

Sweet Almond Oil

-A common skin care oil that is rich in nutrients such as vitamin E, unsaturated fats and essential fatty acids. It has a softening effect on the skin and is good for massage lubrication because it is not absorbed quickly while it is not heavy oil.

Olive Oil

-A heavier oil rich in oleic acid and monounsaturates. Extra virgin olive oil originates from the first pressing of olives and is colored in dark green suggesting the existence of polyphenol antioxidants.

It is suitable for use with dry skin because it helps to balance the cell membrane to improve skin moisture retention. Squalene, a moisturizing andanti-inflammatory agent, also contains olive oil ideally suited for skin conditions such as psoriasis and eczema.

Tamanu Oil

-Tamanu Oil has powerful healing properties in its unique ability to promote new skin tissue development. Oil historically used for skin and mucous membranes by the Polynesians may sustain cuts, burns, skin cracks, slices, dry skin, and wounds.

Tamanu is used for beauty procedures, moderate antibiotics and anti-inflammatory behaviors 2. It is therefore used in defensive as well as regenerative products for restoring the appearance of the skin.

Primrose Evening Oil

-Primrose Evening Oil (EPO) is a precious source of gamma linoleic acid, an essential fatty acid with a strong anti-inflammatory effect. Useful for dry, impaired, sensitive skin EPO helps maintain normal functions of the skin barrier. It is also topically effective for psoriasis and eczema.

Rosehip Oil

-Rosehip oil is very fine with up to 80% essential fatty acid content and is absorbed very quickly by the skin. Rosehip encourages skin regeneration and repair and is known for its skin benefits, particularly in the treatment of scars and burns. It is also renowned for its rehydration and for the treatment of dry, aged and wrinkled skin.

Jojoba Oil

-In fact, rather than an oil, Jojoba oil is very thin and easily absorbed into the skin. It is light and non-greasy and is ideal for serums and creams. Jojoba resembles skin sebum closely and is therefore helpful to skin and scalp disorders, including psoriasis and eczema. It is moisturizing, soothing and ideal for all skin types with outstanding emollient properties.

Cocoon Oil

–One of the toughest and most durable oils, cocoon is suitable for the application of hair and body. It is suitable for dry and rough skin with moisturizing and softening properties. Coconut oil also has cooling properties and is therefore useful for goods after sun treatment 1.

Avocado Oil

-Strong in color and dour, avocado oil is not appropriate for everybody in the skin. It is rich in lecithin, vitamin D, E and A however in its unrefined form and offers useful sun protection and skin nutrition. Avocado oil is good for drying skins.

Sea Buckthorn Oil

-Bright color orange, Sea Buckthorn Oil is high in beta carotene, with Rose Hip only in vitamin C. It is also very high in fatty acids. A rich mix of nutrients ensures that the base oil in your skin is extremely beneficial. It's easy to absorb and effective for all skin types with hydrating, anti-inflammatory and restore properties.

CHAPTER 20

Simple DIY Skin Care Remedies

It can be a little difficult to keep your skin clean. People sometimes abuse their skin unintentionally without realizing it. There are several brand name cleansers, toners, moisturizers and anti-aging products that lead to the degradation of skin.

If you see many of these over - the-counter products, your skin will feel dull, dry and flaccid and will never produce long-term results. Most products cause significant breakouts because most of the counter stuff is designed solely to protect you from sunburn and nothing else.

The other explanation is the chemicals used in the manufacture of the goods. Reading the ingredients closely on the bottles, some of the same ingredients are used for making cleaning products, bleaches and skin-free disinfectants. This is where unintended abuse occurs, and we exploit it further by assuming it will be fixed with the covering of our bodies.

The target should not be just a skin that looks great, but a healthy skin. Below are a few of my own at-home DIY skin care methods and tricks that can help you achieve the objective of healthy skin and radiant healthy glow.

Cleansing

The washing of your face is very necessary. Especially before bed and when you wake up first. Most skin face washers and cleansers contain very dangerous ingredients such as sodium lauryl sulfate and ammonium lauryl sulfate. Sulfates are tensioners which are used as purifiers to remove oil from the skin but are too heavy and dehydrate the body.

If you've ever wondered why you can't get rid of the dry skin, this is probably the reason. A blend of baking soda and witch hazel is one of my favorite home-made cleansers. Mix and add a small amount of water to make a good paste.

Stretch the skin uniformly and wash with gentle circular movement. Baked soda is a natural antibiotic that cures the fungal infections underlying it. It can also slowly remove acne scars and improve acne damage healing. It is also the largest weapon against bacteria, blackheads and inflammation.

Hazel from witch is a natural astringent. It helps reduce the likelihood of inflammation and its strong anti-inflammatory properties are excellent to kill bacteria that develop under pores before they even start.

Not only is a very easy face-washing combo of backing soda and witch hazel very successful. You have to cleanse your skin every day. That's the law. For those who use make up on a daily basis, cleaning is especially necessary. Only do it. Do it.

Dead skin cells stack on the skin surface and look dull and dry. Dead skin cells play a major role in blocking pores. It is essential to exfoliate because it removes dead cells of the skin which obstruct the skin and uncovers new cells.

This opens up the way for hydrating products to penetrate deeper into the skin, making them more effective. You don't have to buy expensive exfoliating products to do the job. You can whip a simple homemade exfoliant that just as easily scrub off those dead skin cells. Bar none of the best are oatmeal exfoliants.

Oatmeal is filled with antioxidants and anti-inflammatory compounds and is considered to provide relief from scratching, snapping and other small skin irritations, including skin calming properties, such as moisturizing dry skin.

Honey provides a natural antibacterial and curative agent that calms and clarifies the skin. Coconut oil is a natural skin food. You just have to blend them together to create a nice mixture and spread easily on your face. Allow the mask to sit about 10 minutes before thorough washing.

The above exfoliant and cleaner recipes are only two of my favorites. There are other variations of recipes you should crochet. Almond oil and sugar, as well as avocado, salt and lemon juice are a great softening agent. All these ingredients form fantastic exfoliate recipes that wash all the dead cells free.

Be mindful that only 1-2 days per week must be exfoliated. Excessive use of exfoliants will remove the skin and make it red and even rash. If you have skin rash or sunburn, do not exfoliate. Cleansers and exfoliants are not similar. Please don't try to swap one with the other. In short, the skin will look fresh and healthy in a daily exfoliation routine.

Moisturize Moisturizing is the main part of the washing of healthy skin. You must hydrate at least twice a day every day. Night and morning. Water is the best moisturizer for the skin. You should not only drink much of it, but also spray your skin every day. Air is preferred for Lukewarm.

Water supplies organic food and hydration for your skin. You can do that by using moisturizers both day and night to keep your skin hydrated and comfortable. If, like me, you don't have the skin that swallows oil like big fish, you should whip up a homemade moisturizer vitamin E, using Aloe Vera plant gel, and shea butter.

Good skin care needs to be such a complex task to achieve a safe and radiant glow. You don't have to spend much money to afford it, either. Certain of the best medications and skin care can be done safely at home by using items right in your cupboards and fridges.

CHAPTER 21

Pay Attention to Skin Care Products Ingredients

Did you know that certain skin care products are not cosmetics, actually? In fact, some skin-care ingredients will change the structure of the skin more than you initially agreed.

It is important to pay attention to the ingredient labels to protect your skin. Some skin care products are laced with harmful chemicals that actually damage your skin. The problem is that it takes some research to find out whether or not a product harms your skin.

Those products that claim to reduce lines, change wrinkles or alter your face can cause a lot of damage. In reality, the government considers different products to be a drug because they contain a lot of harsh chemicals.

Even more fearful than that some products for skin care may actually ruin your skin, is that certain products are not even considered medicines even if they have ingredients that alter the skin. These products are often referred to as "cosmeceutical" skin care products.

Cosmeceutical products actually change the biological make-up of your skin. In short, these products will do much more than alter your skin's look. If you don't want to use skin damaging chemicals, it is best to buy natural skin products.

Skin care can be quite complicated as there are so many competing points of view. Many people will tell you to buy cosmetics, while others are resistant to any type of skin care product. So, what should you do?

You can start by looking for skin care products that contain only ingredients that you can pronounce. This may seem silly, but you shouldn't put the names of the ingredients on your skin if you can't tell them.

First, make sure you just buy natural skin care products. Also, normal means a lot of different things in the skin care industry. Stick with the ingredients you know, or take the time to look for ingredients you don't know about.

Most goods on the market claim to transform your appearance. Nonetheless, many of these products do not work... and most of them can potentially destroy your skin If a product promises to change your appearance, make sure that they do not actually alter the structure of your skin!

Elasticity of the skin is the one thing that keeps the skin from shrinking and falling. When you constantly apply a substance that eats away at the elasticity of your skin, your skin may no longer be normal. Remove any skin care product that may well damage your skin.

Once the skin loses its elasticity, it is difficult to recover. The best way to ensure that you have fresh, radiant skin for years to come is by using natural products that do not harm your skin. Be mindful about what you put on your skin-you only have one chance of handling your skin correctly.

CHAPTER 22

Skin Care Advice For Optimum Skin Care

The advice on skin care merit gold when it applies all natural skin care products to the customer. Healthy and radiant skin, rather than synthetic products, can be accomplished by natural skin care products and organic facial care products. Take the time to search for guidance on skin care to ensure it is fact-based, rather than speculation.

Organic facial moisturizers, lotions and sugars in department and drugstores across the country are increasingly visible.

Consumers are skin-care educated and interested in their products ' ingredients more than in past years. In the organic face care and skin care industry in general, the consumer demand for safer products has been fulfilled by providing a wide variety of products that suit almost every budget.

There's a lot of hype about all natural skin care products. So, what advice can you really believe on skin care?

If you trust what you hear and read, it is important to remember that you are doing your own research. Each customer should be aware of the skin healthy ingredients. Once you buy the labels on your skin care products, make sure they contain natural ingredients.

Which ingredients should be used in your skin care products? Organic face care products and other skin care products, including lotions, serums, cosmetics, creams and shampoos, are intended to contain only holistic and non-synthetic ingredients.

When you apply lotion or other skin care products to your skin, about 60 percent of the ingredients in your skin and bloodstream are absorbed. It is therefore perfectly logical that the ingredients should be normal and therefore not harmful to our bodies.

Remember that advice on skin care from all directions in the form of marketing campaigns may come to you. Be educated in your skin and be prepared to choose the best ingredients for your organic facial care and skin care products.

Vitamin E is a powerful antioxidant that helps the skin resist aging. Vitamin E is effective in reducing the appearance of fine lines, smile lines and skin wrinkles. This vital ingredient defies the free radicals of the air through skin protection and healthy luminosity.

Jojoba oil is another holistic ingredient in all natural skin care and organic products. It is essentially a vegetable oil, but the very structure of the oil in the skin, called sebum, is an ideal moisturizer for the skin. Hydrated skin naturally looks younger and healthier.

In and around the eye area, many women show their age. A good choice is organic facial care products containing grapefruit oil. Evidence has shown that grapefruit oil protects the skin around the eyes, significantly reducing the development of wrinkles and fine lines.

And you got it there. Please note that advice on skin care should be considered if it leads you to all natural and organic skin care. These are the goods with natural and balanced ingredients that will give you results.

Problems with sensitive skin include redness, swelling, rashes, dry skin, discomfort and general skin irritation. Sensitive skin can be a problem for people with different types of skin, including oily skin.

Here are 5 things you should do for the best treatment of your skin.

1. Have a test for allergy. There are various allergies that cause skin problems and it is always worthwhile seeing if you can develop a particular skin condition. If you can decide exactly what causes (or may not) the problem, something can be done about it.

2. Avoid large-scale skin care products. The large-scale skin care items are riddled with additives that can cause people with sensitive skin types to suffer. Regrettably, the FDA does not really regulate skin care ingredients, many with suspected or known ingredients that cause cancer and other conditions, including skin problems.

It is ironic that many anti-aging and skin care products brands create skin p and other health issues. The skin doesn't approve of artificial chemicals, and many people will find that different skin reactions are the result.

An event to think about. There are a number of common parabens induced chemicals that are commonly used as preservatives in big brand-name skin care products. Parabens are classified as hazardous in the cosmetic database, two as a significant risk of at least 7 or 8 in scale 1 to 10.

Parabens can cause skin problems themselves, and this is only one example. There are many ingredients like this used in skin care products that can make your skin responsive to otherwise healthy.

3. And with cosmetics it's almost the same. Here is an example. Here is an example. Recent tests have demonstrated lead in more than 50 percent of large brand lipsticks including some ones you can use now. Stop cosmetics for big brands.

And an allergy test may well indicate that your cosmetic or skin care so anti-aging products have an allergy to one or more of the ingredients.

For those who require high-quality sensitive skin care without large brand cosmetics and skin care, it may be enough to reverse their skin problems.

4. Once clothes and other household items are cleaned, using low irritant detergents. Washing detergents can also cause skin problems for people with sensitive skin and normal healthy skin.

For instance, if you wash your pillow cases and sheets in a washing detergent with allergens or irritants on your skin, spend 8 hours lying on that pillow case with your face and causing problems themselves.

So stop anything with fragrances, like detergents. Cosmetics and skin care products are included. Fragrances also have their issues, sadly. Fragrances are chemicals which can cause skin issues, just like some other gross (and unregulated) skin care ingredients and cosmetic products.

5. Look for some natural cosmetics and skin care and anti-aging products.

Excellent natural cosmetics and products for skin care are available. They are manufactured by small, not household names niche companies.

Many businesses are committed to making high-quality skin care, anti-aging products and cosmetics suitable for optimum skin sensitivity. We are usually highly competitive in price because these businesses don't spend a lot on TV advertising.

And the products usually do what they say, contrary to those big brand names you see on the shelves of your stores, which are to be avoided.

Their products are made with natural, safe, non-allergenic plant ingredients, and those companies are as committed to safety as their products are to quality. And their skin care products are perfect for people with skin problems.

Good skin quality is a major problem for people with sensitive skin. Besides the blurry redness and dryness, discomfort and itching can make you mad. For these men, sensitive skin care is a big problem.

There are 5 things that you can do to fix the problem if you have serious skin issues. Do all this and you may well find that your skin issues are just gone. Of course, it is not guaranteed, but this is the best place to start optimally sensitive skin care.

CHAPTER 23

Homemade Skin Care: 7 Tips for Creating Flawless Radiant Skin

If you plan to make your own home-made skin care remedies, here are some tips on how to use them. When it comes to any health problem, it is always best to start with a daily routine. When it comes to personal skin treatments, you need to develop definite healthy habits. Use these helpful home-made tips for skin care to get you started.

Exfoliate Every Evening

Make sure you exfoliate every night after you meet your nose. Make sure you use a good wash. If you haven't made an exfoliating recipe yet, only sugar or oatmeal can be quickly exfoliated. It's just as fast. Not a bad idea to try when you're running out of business stuff.

Using face masks

This move is one that many of us, including me, are guilty of ignoring. Maybe we don't want to look stupidly in front of wives or babies, but these consequences are necessary to forget.

Create face masks if you can use one of the best tools to keep your skin look beautiful. Not only will the skin look and feel better, but at the end of a long day, it is a great way to relax. When I want to rest and see the end of the day, I do this.

I didn't use moisturizer when I was younger and now I know the value of using one. I don't really use moisturizer. Why does it matter so much?

Okay, mostly because your skin is hydrating. Most skin care experts recommend using moisturizers at night to allow undisturbed skin to penetrate. You also recommend that you treat the skin with alpha hydroxylic acids, vitamins A or C, and then add the hydrating agent. It's absorbed into the skin in this way.

If you use home-made natural ingredients, treat your skin kindly. Treat your skin with respect. When you clean just because we call facial scrubs, don't be rough on your face.

You don't wash your skin like the floor of the bathroom. You will lower the risk of harming it and having unwanted wrinkles, but take into account the implications of being too rough on your face.

Do not try to stay indoors like a vampire, but you have to take the necessary precautions, particularly if you sunbathe. Take the right lotions on your hands. You may also wish to avoid the tanning salon since your smooth, brown skin prematurely increases the chances of wrinkles. Worse still, it can lead to cancer.

Eat fresh foods

What you put in your mouth does indeed show in your skin's health. Most people avoid chocolate because acne has worsened. But this is a good reason enough to stay away, right? It should not be shocking that proper nutrition actually improves the appearance of your skin.

Drink plenty of water

Keeping your skin hydrated helps keep your skin safe. This increases your organ functioning and because your skin is your largest organ, it only makes sense how it can support your teint. Many health professionals recommend that you drink at least eight to 10 glasses of water a day.

Through setting up regular skin routines, you open up opportunities for health and beauty.

One of the reasons why I engaged in the development of natural skin care recipes was because I wanted to improve the consistency of my skin and relax and treat myself to a much needed treatment.

You will care for your skin because it is a symbol that you have a healthy life. Follow these ideas before you go to bed, so that you can know more about natural, herbal treatments that can lead to a healthier look.

CHAPTER 24

Homemade Skin Lightener For Permanent And Natural Whitening Skin

Using a natural lightener is a sweetest way to avoid the harsh chemicals in bleaching agents and other skin lightening creams. Below are some of the best natural skin lightning receptions that you can build from the comfort of your house to a beautiful and rising teint.

With the pollutants and the harsh rays of the sun and skin, most people are full of age, dark arms and legs, and uneven skin tones. The main reason is because the melanin content of the skin is hyperpigmented or compounded.

Honey and almond:

As honey was a skin emollient agent, often used for humectating and emollient purposes, amond is also one of the best whitening agents in various skin care products. Why are you using them?

Take 1 teaspoon of honey plus ½ almond powder tablespoon and 1 tsp of lemon. Allow it to be rinsed with water for 15 minutes afterwards. This method works well to eliminate a tan and gives a beautiful, shiny teint.

Milk and Almond:

All you have to do is grind some almonds and mix with fresh milk to apply this process. Apply the mixture on your face for 15 minutes. Let it proceed. Then wash your face with cold water. The regular use of this recipe guarantees a strong teint.

Lemon Juice and Rose Water: Lemon juice is the key to restore a great teint. It's a dark skin lightener. Using it with rose water is easy to get fair complexion. And lovely skin.

The only part is that you don't have to lie down and wait until your mask dries away. You can only submit and maintain your daily routine.

The application of sandalwood powder mixed with turkey juice, lemon juice and tomato juice results in better, more beautiful, lighter, brighter, and even skin tones.

Another method is by mixing 3 tsp of sandalwood powder with 3 tabs of rose water and wearing this face mask for at least 20 minutes.

Tomato and oatmeal:

Oatmeal is the unique exfoliating agent for slugging your dried skin. Applying oatmeal, tomato juice and curd, leaving it on in cold water for 20 minutes, can help to set off that horrible skin tanning.

Yogurt help:

Take yoghurt and mix with papaya or strawberries, add one tablespoon of blackberry sauce, one tablespoon of blackberry sauce and 1 tablespoon of olive oil and spread the mixture for 20 mins before you clean it off.

<u>Use of Gram Meal:</u>

In a small mixing bowl, mix 2 tablespoons of flour with a little turmeric and add 2 teaspoons of milk to it. Then add the mixture and let it run for 15 minutes until cold water purifies it.

You should be aware that all the home-made skin lighteners may not necessarily be the quickest options there, but they definitely differ in your skin tone and complexion when used regularly. With these techniques, certain hard bleaching agents will not be required to damage your skin.

CHAPTER 25

Homemade Skin Exfoliator To Remove Dead Skin Cells

An exfoliation can quickly remove the outer layer of the oldest and dead skin cells. Thanks to exfoliation, skin is healthy, eliminates acne breakouts and also unblocks pores.

Easily prepare your own skin exfoliator at home. There are many ways to prepare exfoliators at home. You should prepare skin exfoliator at home, using natural ingredients, to care for your skin naturally. Below, some of the best ways to prepare skin exfoliator at home.

1. The homemade skin exfoliator can be prepared by adding one tsp of sugar, one tsp of olive oil, one tsp glycerin and a few drops of patchouli oil. Then massage this mixture softly into your body with circular motion.

Wash this after a moment. This scrub is very good for dry skin.

2. Mix one tablespoon of baking soda and one tablespoon of your favorite cleanser or face lotion. Gently wash your face by circularly rubbing this mixture. Rinse and apply moisturizer.

3. Mixing baking soda with aloe vera can also make a homemade skin exfoliator. Create a smooth paste, mixing one tablespoon of baking soda with enough aloe vera juice or gel.

If the paste is too wet, it's easy to add some baking powder. Using new aloe vera or even bottled. Scrub this mixture in circular motion for 1-2 minutes. Rinse, tone, and moisturize your face.

4. The home-made exfoliator can be combined with one tsp of honey, one tsp of salt. Add few drops of patchouli oil in these ingredients. Mix ingredients well. Gently clean this mixture upon wetting.

Scrub the mixture circularly and wash clean. This exfoliator is very useful for oily skin. It's salt and honey scrub. A common skin exfoliator used at home.

5. Another easy exfoliator is prepared using gram flour and moong dal. It's an easy wash, too. To prepare it, mix one tsp gram flour and one tsp moong dal. Using milk and rose water to combine these ingredients. This scrub is very good for skin combination.

CHAPTER 26

Homemade Potato Masks for Skin Care

You eat potato almost everyday. Boiled or fried, baked or mashed-potato is very tasty, and everyone knows this fact. But not everyone knows potato is a wonderful product for cosmetic face masks.

Indeed, it's the ultimate cosmetic product. It's safe, cheap and effective for skin care! The explanation is potato tubers ' chemical composition, which includes many substances that are beneficial for the skin.

Next, it's vitamin C. This participates in collagen synthesis—a natural product that gives skin firmness and elasticity, protecting skin from premature aging and adverse external influences.

Specific proteins exist in potato tubers, which enable the epidermal cell regeneration process and facilitate wound and crack healing. These minerals as zinc and copper smooth slight wrinkles.

You'll need 2 tablespoons of potato starch and warm water. Put starch in a tub. Garnish with warm water, blend carefully. Apply greasy cream to face and neck. Apply starch mixture with wide soft brush. Do not add the mask around the eyes and the neck front surface. Soften the starch mass with wet compress after 20 minutes, rinse with warm water.

Good advice!

Potto starch mask effectively tightens pores, improves local blood circulation, and smoothes. But it's driing the surface. Therefore, having this mask really often isn't recommended.

To make your hands soft you'll need 2-3 potatoes, 3-4 tablespoons warm milk, water. Boil onions, peel and mash. Mix carefully with milk. Add mashed potatoes to hands and hold for about half an hour on the surface.

Good advice! Potato mash envelope will also help you remove skin irritation.

1. Moistening potato and milk lotion

4 tablespoons of potato decoction and 5 tablespoons of milk.

Directions

Cook potatoes. Take decoction, wait until it cools, then blend with milk. Pour the mixture into container and refrigerate. Pre-use shake vigorously. Using gentle circular motions to lotion your face and keep for 10-15 minutes. Cover with paper towel.

2. Oily skin lotion

Directions

1/4 cup raw potato juice and 1/4 cup tomato juice. Peel, squeeze and pour the resulting juice into the container. Do the same with tomatoes. Add two juices of vegetables. Wash face and neck skin with cotton pad in prepared lotion. Render this morning and evening practice.

CHAPTER 27

Benefits of Using Strawberries As a Homemade Natural Skin Care Product

Strawberries are not only delicious fruits you eat fresh or as toppings on cheesecakes and other desserts, they are also a perfect ingredient for homemade face washing and body scrubbing. As a fruit, strawberries have many health benefits for the body, such as antioxidant properties and folic acid.

In Roman times, used strawberries with their medicinal properties. These have more vitamin C than other fruits, making them a viable alternative for lemons and oranges. Yet strawberries have all the skin's natural ingredients that can be healthy.

Everything strawberries can do for your skin has an acidic property that can take all those dead skin cells off your skin. This property makes strawberries perfectly natural.

It's also salicylic acid that can fight blackheads and acne.

So for those who struggle to manage acne and blemishes on their bodies, strawberries can be just the kind of fruit you need to eat, and the kind of natural food you can turn into a beauty product.

Besides these attractive qualities, strawberries can also become a natural skin care regimen, as they have natural ingredients that can make the skin lighter. This is good news for those who want a lighter skin tone. Instead of buying beauty products worth $100, you should make your own strawberry scrub. Wait a few weeks for the amazing result.

Strawberries also have antiseptic properties. That's why they've been used in medicinal days. They include properties and natural chemicals that protect the body against bacteria and other diseases.

If you have freckles on your face or your entire body, you should patch strawberry juice. Squeeze the juice out of the strawberry and cover it with a cotton ball. It can also remove possible causes of acne including dust and allergens.

It's a wonder why people spend hundreds of dollars for facial scrub at a salon or dermatologist's clinic. You can recover oily or dry skin by simply mashing and adding strawberry. A mashed strawberry will stay 15-20 minutes on your nose. Wash it with lukewarm water and see results in daily facial weeks.

Blend sunflower, olive or corn oil with mashed strawberry before applying the mixture to your skin.

CHAPTER 28

Secrets For Making Your Own Homemade Skin Care Recipes

Skin care is the most important part of a beauty routine. Your skin gives a glow to your appearance, and care should be taken when applying any creams, moisturizers, sunscreens, facials or masks. So long as they're made of natural and organic materials, it's good for your skin.

You'll find from our pages a host of details about using natural and organic skin care products. You can also use the information to make your own skin care recipe, which is genuinely nice to your teint regardless of skin tone.

Lemon juice, yogurt, lavender, almonds, olive oil, milk, orange peel, sugar, grenade juice, turmeric powder, salt and honey all suit our exclusive skin care recipes. Our insightful pages will help you prepare these recipes yourself, using a mix of natural and herbal ingredients.

The recipe you prepare is cheap and safe to use. No adverse effect on the skin, giving it a natural glow and softness. The skin won't have as many free-radicals and will promote skin cell growth.

Preparing these skin care recipes won't be a Herculean task if you follow the instructions carefully given in the web ages. The more you browse the internet, the more you get about different uses of natural and organic materials.

Trying it at home will be a fun and enjoyable experience, and you can do it while you're busy with your cooking recipes, so take care of proportions. You can use various items to measure, create and store recipes such as cups, bottles, jars and bowls that are available in your kitchen. You will also need a strainer and blender as part of your kitchen tools collection.

The simple process by which the skin care formula can be prepared includes peeling, mashing, and straining, which need no expertise. The more you involve yourself; the more you enjoy.

Sometimes you'll feel like a laboratory testing scientist. Inventing a new and original skin care recipe will get you happy, and you'll be inspired to scream "Eureka!" Once you're able to prepare your own skin care recipes, you can start improvising by learning about each ingredient's qualities.

So do away with inorganic and artificial skin care lotions, creams, masks, and moisturizers that are your skin's real enemies. You won't look back after picking up the secrets of preparing skin care recipes and having wonderful results.

Sharing your thoughts and experiences will certainly enlighten your knowledge and help you become your own beautician.

You can now share your skin care experience and even consider selling it under your own brand name! Make your skin as attractive as ever. Look at you and think about your skin care secrets.

Make Homemade Beauty Skin Care Products Beauty products need not be costly.

Yeah, some of the best skin care remedies can be found inside your refrigerator. Actually, I'm not thinking about the ultra-expensive dermatologist-prescribed treatments you need to refrigerate before using.

I'm talking about products that can be used to treat beauty on your face. Such natural beauty skin care products operate as well as store-bought cosmetics, but are much cheaper.

Mashed fruits mixed with other foods in your kitchen make a good facial scrub or mask. To make your own facial scrub, take a fistful or grape and pound it to a pulp. Carefully remove skins before pouring one tablespoon of almond flavor into the grape juice and pulp mixture. Apply the mixture directly to your nose.

It can be made of a spoonful of sugar and several drops of olive oil. If you want, add more to exfoliate your entire body.

A mixture of crushed bananas and honey is a perfect skin care product. Mash a banana and mix it with 3 honey spoons to make your own mask.

Adding half a cup of honey to your bathwater is excellent beauty treatments that can enhance skin texture, making it feel cleaner and softer.

Many skin care products, whether handmade or sold, use aloe vera. It can be used as an astringent to combat oily skin. Even, Aloe Vera can be massaged to make your crowning glory smoother and safer. Just make sure your 15-minute rinse off.

Baking soda is another natural skin care product that cannot only clear blackheads from your face, but also buildup your hair. Combine just as much baking soda and water together to make a solution. Apply it to your face and hair, rinse after 15 minutes. You'll be shocked at what your skin and hair can do.

CHAPTER 29

Tips For High Quality Natural Skin Care

If we want some information about something, the net is an excellent source of information. Under the light, we can find various details about anything like gardening, cooking recipes and even beauty tips.

When it comes to beauty tips, however, verify the information you gathered from the internet. Compare the guides and ideas below and choose what you think will work best for you.

You must be very careful to try internet beauty tips. Remember some issues before carrying out the tips you've heard. Good advice usually includes alerts, such as ensuring you don't have allergies to certain substances and much more.

Determine the actual limitations of beauty tips right after. Many of these tips discuss health advice concerning drinking fluids, especially water.

We all know water is good for us; however, you need to remember that not all people are built for the same liquid level. Toddlers, athletes, and those with kidney disease almost all have unique factors in how much drinking water is required.

Doing something excessively will create trouble. Of example, exfoliating is mostly recommended for people with no specific skin conditions, like every other skin care procedure, the accuracy of exfoliation can vary depending on skin sensitivity and dryness.

In terms of home-made skin care remedies, you need to think about the ingredients you use. Apple cider vinegar is an illustration of several home-made health and beauty cures, such as pimples.

Remember, though, that apple cider vinegar has high acetic chemical content? Using apple cider vinegar containing a lot of acetic acid will potentially damage the skin, making it melt away.

Besides home-made skin care remedies, you also need to look at the anti-aging product components before use. This is a good way to prevent more harm to your skin, as we all know that not all products on the market are safe and effective. Not all of these products contain all natural ingredients, so you need to read the product label before you purchase it.

If you're still unsure or confused, ask your own skin doctor or dermatologist for advice. These are the types of people who know these things. They'll give you tips to match your skin type. Until testing any product, make sure it's safe and reliable.

If a certain product offers you to look twenty years younger in a moment, think about it well because it takes a lot of energy, time and money to obtain a healthy, smooth and younger face. Note that these are cosmetics firms ' marketing strategies, so don't be fooled.

Skin care products are top sellers in the skin care industry. More and more people are recognizing that the additives used in big brand name skin care products are not safe for us or our skin and shifting to natural alternatives for skin care products, hair care products and cosmetics.

Although the best natural skin care and anti-aging products are spectacularly effective, more can be achieved than using organic skin care products.

1. <u>Boost diet.</u>

Our diet affects our entire body and our skin. Our skin is like any other organ in our body, and like other organs our skin can get unhealthy from an unhealthy diet. But as everyone sees your eyes, a poor diet is highly visible.

It refers to all skin types, whether you have oily skin, dry skin, or skin type, poor diet can affect your skin's health and appearance. Avoid burgers and pizzas for fruit and vegetables, and your skin will look much better, and you'll be healthier.

2. <u>Avoid cosmetics and skin care products.</u>

Such products, including items like hair treatments, hair removal procedures, famous cosmetics, many facial and body care products, and more, contain chemicals that can both damage your health and harm your skin. Unfortunately, skin care products and cosmetics can cause skin problems. Junk the brand-name products.

The author's personal experience of this. Her ballet studio gave my young daughter conventional makeup for her first ballet concert a few years ago, and immediately broke out in a nasty skin reaction. We use our own (natural) cosmetics for her now, and there was no repeat.

3. Stick to a regular exercise schedule.

Exercise increases blood circulation, which is good for your skin and your whole body. Exercise has so many benefits it's hard to know where to start, including better skin health.

4. Consider plenty of beneficial essential oils in your diet.

It includes omega-3, which comes from eating fish and other plants. Omega 3 is good for your skin and health.

You can get omega 3 from good (natural) supplements, but just figure out which foods contain omega 3 and eat them if you're on a budget. Do some research and find a good source of beneficial omega-3 oil, and include it regularly in your diet.

5. Drink lots of water. Your body and skin must stay hydrated. If you don't drink water, this will affect your overall health and safety. Water is essential to much of your body, including skin health.

8. Start exfoliation of dry hair.

Sounds complicated, but exfoliation uses a smooth, dry brush to gently clean your skin. Why would you clean your skin? Dry brush exfoliation helps remove dead skin cells on the surface of our skin.

And not just brush the skin on your nose, you should brush your entire body. Gently brushing from your feet to your chin in small circles. Dry brush exfoliation also helps improve skin circulation and lymph circulation.

7. Know your face.

The first thing to do is to decide your skin type, because it will determine the products you choose and the regular regimen you follow. No one product would fit every skin type. Your form is defined as dry, oily, or combination. Look for products specific to your particular type.

8. Clean skin twice daily.

Every day we're exposed to dust, free radicals, and toxins outside that can damage our bodies.

While our skin doesn't look "dirty," we must be sure to clean daily, and the recommended amount is twice a day. Using lukewarm water instead of very hot or very cold water when bathing or washing your hair, as both can also harm the skin.

9. Gently treat your skin.

For your skin, scrubbing or exfoliating too often is not pleasant. Never rub, but gently massage the cleanser with upward circular motions. When you age, skin loses its elasticity and rubbing or pulling it can cause the skin to sink.

10. Use humidifier. Dry skin looks bad because it doesn't get the right nutrients. The dryness can actually cause the skin to crack, resulting in an unattractive look. Choose the best moisturizer for your skin type and apply it over damp skin. Just make sure it's a good quality product providing the necessary nutrients for best skin care.

11. NEVER use face body wash.

This form of soap is used below the face. Only use cleansers made for the face because they are easier on your skin.

12. Use Sunscreen.

This cannot be stressed enough. Use sunscreen protects the skin from sun's harmful UV rays. You may think if it's cloudy you don't need sunscreen, but that's not true. Skin cancer can be caused by UV rays, so don't ignore this very critical skin care tip.

13. Exercise and sleep comfortably.

Both are important for healthy skin and overall. Sleeplessness and lack of exercise are both sources of skin loss and wrinkles. All exercise and sleep will help you overcome any stress in your life that makes you look better.

14. Ignore skin conditions.

Pay attention to your skin, and if you find any irregularities, see your dermatologist immediately. Once you start self-diagnosing and treating yourself, it's best to find out what the disorder is, which could lead to more issues.

15. Try beating pain.

Although we all have stress in our lives, there are ways to reduce it. Understand that stress is harmful to your health and appearance. It will also harm the skin, so be aware of this and try to do things to help lower your life's stress.

You can do 15 items free to help improve your skin beauty routine. You can save some money, for example, fruits and vegetables are usually cheaper than burgers and pizzas. And if you do these 6 things regularly, they'll boost your skin health over time, and you'll see results. And your body will be grateful with improved overall health.

One final thing. Once you've junked your big brand name skin care products and cosmetics, hair and facial and body care products, consider some high-quality products for natural skin care.

These work better than the big brand names (many of which do nothing at all) and are made from healthy, non-allergenic ingredients. Science seeks solutions to skin aging and skin health, which comes from healthy plant extracts including shea butter and natural keratin.

Conclusion

There are many other ways to take care of your skin's well-being without spending a fortune on any kind of expensive wash. Increasingly, people advocate using the natural alternative with organic ingredients to achieve the desired healthy, beautiful, shiny and flawless skin, especially the face.

But most of us don't study well to really know what "natural" means, what more to understand how the ingredients in the product function.

A number of preservatives and chemicals known as "carcinogens" and "parabens" can affect your skin and overall health and may not get the desired results. Read the ingredients carefully as you would only know if the product is successful or not.

Besides, you need a reasonable awareness of what some of these chemicals do to your health in the long run. Don't be confused by these chemicals ' industrial titles, most are as harmful as they look.

As natural advocates say,' don't put anything on your body you wouldn't want in your body.' Hair shouldn't be viewed like an alien, just place on your hair what you can eat. Treat it right by finding the right beauty ingredients or recipe.

Some well-known natural ingredients are milk, honey, almond, olive oil and witch hazel used for their distinct properties. Such ingredients have been used since ancient times for cleaning and healing purposes (and yes, they are edible too!).

Isn't it frustrating to spend hard-earned money on products that simply don't deliver results they claim? Maybe this isn't the first time it happens? Maybe it's time to go back to basics.

Some of the most popular skin care techniques are all originally natural and organic. Use naturally derived products like milk and honey for home-made natural recipes can be better than store-bought creams, lotions and masks. After all, these recipes were used for hundreds and even thousands of years, back to Cleopatra's day. Her key to smooth, soft skin, for example, indulged in milk baths.

It can be interesting how these all-natural recipes of origin can be so helpful. Compared to costly skin care products, they can stand their ground. These work to improve skin texture and do not include colors, perfume and preservatives.

This helps relax the epidermis and hydrates the skin. We raise skin moisture levels and improve its ability to protect itself against free radicals and toxins. Such benefits are very close to those imported creams, lotions and masks say as products, except home-made skin care is cheap and safe to use.

If you're new to this, I'd suggest a quick Google search online. You will find a wide range of possibilities in natural and organic skin care, and will certainly be overwhelmed by the amount of information. With hundreds or even thousands of recipes to make scrubs, creams and masks, you'll get busy!

When you read the recipes, you'll know that these recipes are simple and straightforward. There are no complex measures, nor do you need expensive tools. Most of the resources you may need include things like a mixer, measuring cups, and a mixing bowl. It's as effortless as it seems!

If you regularly use natural skin care techniques, you will become comfortable and know that you do not need to rely or focus on other people's recipes. You can start preparing your own recipes! Start by using the ingredients, you believe your skin's teint can improve and benefit more.

Natural skin care is so flexible, allowing you space to experiment and develop your own recipes that are best suited to your skin type. It's endless to make new and improved recipes! Be excited about the ingredients you'll hear about and look forward to the best your skin can be!

« If you enjoyed this book, please let me know your thoughts by leaving a short review on Amazon »

Thank You !

Olivia Hann